MRCP PART 2
PREPARATION FOR THE CLINICAL EXAMINATION

Julian A Gray MA MB BS MRCP(UK)

MRC Training Fellow and Honorary Medical Registrar,
MRC Unit and University Department of Clinical Pharmacology,
Radcliffe Infirmary,
Oxford.

Formerly Research Registrar in Neurology,
Regional Neurological Unit,
Royal Surrey County Hospital,
Guildford.

PASTEST SERVICE
KNUTSFORD
ENGLAND

Egerton Court, Parkgate Estate,
Knutsford, Cheshire WA16 8DX
Telephone: 01565 755226

First published 1986
Reprinted 1988
Reprinted 1991
Reprinted 1993
Reprinted 1995

British Library Cataloguing in Publication Data

Gray, Julian A.
MRCP pt. II clinical: a systematic approach to preparing for the long cases, short case and viva : exam technique planning and preparing.

1. Medicine - Problems, exercises, etc.
I. Title
610'.76 R834.5

ISBN 0-906896-45-2

Text prepared by Turner Associates, Congleton, Cheshire.
Phototypeset by Designed Publications using an interface.
Printed by Hobbs The Printers, Totton, Hampshire.

CONTENTS

FOREWORD

It is a great pleasure to write a foreword to this book which I believe will be of much benefit to candidates undertaking the Clinical part of the Membership examination.

I share Dr Gray's view that the examination, while difficult, is a fair test of clinical skills. It has, in fact, been our experience on our clinical course at Guildford that many candidates, although knowledgeable, are poorly prepared when it comes to carrying out a competent physical examination. This particularly applies to the short cases where candidates can easily be faulted on the soundness of the basic techniques which they use in elucidating the required information when under close scrutiny.

It must, of course, be appreciated that no book can be a substitute for good practical experience. Nevertheless, I am firmly of the opinion that this book will be an invaluable aid in the preparation of many candidates for an examination which is a prerequisite for higher training in medicine.

J D Carroll, MD, FRCP, FRCPE, FRCPI
Physician-in-Charge
Regional Neurological Unit
Royal Surrey County Hospital
Guildford
Surrey

INTRODUCTION

The clinical section of the MRCP examination is the part which many candidates fear most and indeed it is here that the majority of failures occur.

All too commonly the candidate has prepared in completely the wrong way. Then, with the added stress of being observed and questioned by eminent physicians, it is only too easy to look uncertain and unprofessional and to utter statements which even to your own ears sound wrong and even ridiculous. This generally ends in a strong desire for the earth to open and swallow you up!

Thus, most candidates fail themselves: a thoroughly miserable experience which can generally be avoided by careful and thoughtful preparation.

This book is not intended to teach you medicine: you should know this already. Instead, it is a guide on how to prepare for, and hence pass, the clinical examination.

ACKNOWLEDGEMENTS

I wish to thank Doctors Andrew Duncombe, Michael Hardman, Desmond Carroll and Colin Forfar for helpful discussions. All responsibility for the accuracy of the text is of course entirely my own.

My thanks are also due to Mrs Tamsin Dunningham for her expert secretarial assistance and to my wife for her patient support.

Note: For the sake of brevity, references to books have been abbreviated in the text to the name of the author, full references being listed on p. 145.

1 : PREPARING FOR THE CLINICAL

General Points

The Clinical part of the MRCP Part II examination is in three parts: the short cases, the long case, and the viva. In general, the short case section is by far the most difficult and accordingly should occupy the bulk of your preparation time. You should devise and commit to memory a scheme for short case examination. Suggested methods for this are set out in Chapters 4, 5 and 6 but they should be modified to your own taste. Most of your practising, however, should be done on the wards seeing patients as you would in the examination.

As early as possible you should team up with a like-minded candidate with whom you get on well. Not only is this more fun than working alone but it is infinitely more effective. This is because of the need to practise in front of an observer. You will be surprised at how much more difficult it is to perform well when being watched, even by someone you know. You must get used to this as early as possible. In my opinion, practising alone is virtually useless.

You should also persuade a registrar or senior registrar with recent experience of the examination to take you round a series of 'unseen' short cases on a regular basis. For maximum benefit, these sessions should be kept as realistic as possible with the 'examiner' behaving in a suitably cool and neutral manner. Any discussion about how you are getting on should be left until the end of the whole session. This will give you experience of the difficulty of seeing several different cases in quick succession and of keeping going even if you have made a mistake.

You must rehearse as frequently as possible, both with your fellow candidate and with your senior colleague(s), beginning *at least* three months before the clinical and not waiting until after the written paper. On occasion you should intersperse your short case sessions with long cases or viva practice; however, unless you find these particularly difficult, you should not spend too much time on them.

Use your polished examination techniques, with no short cuts, in the clinics and on the wards at all times.

With time and perseverance you will start to notice improvement in your performance. This should lead to an increase in your self-confidence: you will not pass the examination without a reasonable amount of this.

Finally, if you are approaching your preparation correctly you should find that you are actually deriving some enjoyment from it. Both the sharpening of your clinical skills and the element of gamesmanship involved can be very stimulating. If you feel miserable *all* the time there must be something fundamentally wrong in your approach!

Equipment to take with you

Before starting your preparation for the long and short cases you should make sure that you possess a complete set of reliable diagnostic instruments. It is not worth economising over this: it is a great advantage in the clinical to be using equipment with which you have practised and feel at home.

I would suggest that you keep the following in your ‘armoury’:

1. Stethoscope
2. Watch with a second hand
3. Ophthalmoscope
4. Pen torch (with new batteries)
5. Tendon hammer, with long handle and *soft* rubber end
6. Red and white hat pins: heads should be 5 mm diameter
7. Tuning fork (128 cps)
8. Cotton wool
9. Orange sticks (for testing plantar responses)
10. Wooden spatulae
11. Tape measure
12. Pocket ruler
13. Pocket-sized reading chart (invaluable for quickly testing visual acuity).

2 : THE VIVA

It is in the clinical part of the MRCP examination that you first come face to face with your examiners. The clinical may begin with either the long and short cases or the viva. In either case, the impression you make is critical to your success. Thus, however much knowledge you have, you may still fail if the examiners feel that your manner and behaviour towards the patients and themselves is not professional and appropriate.

The following points are important both in the viva and in the rest of the clinical:

Communicate clearly with your examiners

Aim to hold their attention and to interest them. Speak audibly and clearly, looking the examiners in the eye. If you do not understand a question, say so at once. Do not hesitate for more than a few seconds before replying to a question; to do so gives an air of uncertainty which could lessen the examiners' confidence in you. Similarly, you should avoid words such as *possibly* and *I think*.

Always avoid using abbreviations such as JVP etc.

Be honest in your ignorance

Remember that this is not a specialist examination. Provided that you have read widely for the previous parts of the examination, you are unlikely to be asked to discuss subjects about which you are totally ignorant. Even so, the subject matter is so large that you are bound to come across blank spots from time to time. Do not feel too upset if this happens during the examination; you are not expected to know everything! The important thing is to admit this at once. Unless the area of ignorance is one of a basic nature, this will not necessarily be held against you. If it concerns a difficult management question, it is as well to say that you would normally obtain advice from an expert.

For example, you might be asked how you would manage a glutethimide overdose. Although you may not know the specific management the examiners are likely to be satisfied if you reply that you would institute the emergency care of any overdose patient (e.g. maintenance of airway, support of circulation, consideration of gastric lavage, etc.) and then take specialist advice by telephoning the Poisons Information Centre. This indicates that you are practical and safe and is far better than just saying "I don't know" or concocting a fictitious answer.

The questions asked in the viva tend to take one of three forms:

A. **Questions about the management of medical conditions.** These can relate to either outpatient or emergency medicine. The question is often phrased so as to place the candidate in the clinical situation. For example, you might be asked the following: "A woman comes to your clinic complaining that hair is growing on her face. What are you going to do?" Another example could be: "Your houseman telephones you from Casualty to say that he has just admitted a patient with a blood glucose of 40. How will you proceed?"

B. **Questions testing general medical knowledge.** The scope here is obviously vast. However, it is worth remembering that it is common for questions to be asked on applied science, such as the mechanism of drug actions and interactions, and elementary clinical physiology, such as respiratory function tests.

C. **Questions about topical issues** e.g. alcohol, drug abuse, antiviral therapy.

To prepare for the viva you should continue with some general reading although this must not be allowed to detract from the time spent on preparing for the cases. If you have made notes for the multiple choice and written sections, you should re-read them. You must also study the leading articles in the Lancet and British Medical Journal for at least six months before the examination. Many of the examiners also read the Quarterly Journal of Medicine, so it is worth looking through this as well.

Turning to the actual viva there are a few general points to remember about answering questions. Firstly, if asked to talk about a large subject, e.g. the harmful effects of alcohol, you will give a much better impression if you can *structure your answer* in an orderly manner. Sticking to our example, you might say "I normally divide these into physical, psychological and social effects". This also gives the impression that you have considered the topic before and that you have organised your thoughts about it. Secondly, when asked about your management of any condition, always start by emphasising that you would *take a thorough history and perform a full examination.* You will never lose by saying this as it shows you are aware of their importance in good clinical practice. Thirdly, *always mention common conditions before rare ones.* Contrary to popular opinion, the Membership examination is more concerned with basic general medicine than with rare and exotic conditions: if asked the causes of pleural effusions you will not create the right impression by mentioning Meig's syndrome first!

The Viva

The two examiners will each ask you questions for ten minutes. At the end of this period, remember to thank the examiners and leave graciously.

The following is a selection of topics which is intended to give an idea of the range of questions which can be asked in a viva. It is by no means intended as an exhaustive list since there is of course no limit to the number of possible questions. Topical subjects have not been included as they change rapidly and in general can be predicted from recent leading articles.

Discuss the management of:

Atypical pneumonia, especially Legionnaire's disease
Cardiac arrhythmias
Chloroquine-resistant malaria
Exercise-induced asthma
Exophthalmos
Gall stones
Gout
Hyperlipidaemia
Infective endocarditis
Migraine
Myasthenia gravis
Obesity
Paget's disease
Parkinsonism (including the "on-off" effect)
Portal hypertension
Trigeminal neuralgia
Ulcerative colitis/Crohn's disease.

Clinical approach questions: of the type "How would you manage a patient with.....................?"

14-year-old male presenting with eneuresis
15-year-old female presenting with haematuria
15-year-old boy with hypertension
21-year-old female referred to outpatient clinic because of hirsutism
30-year-old man referred because of asymptomatic proteinuria discovered during insurance examination
60-year-old male with a haemoglobin of 19g.
14-year-old boy with short stature
24-year-old female referred to outpatient clinic because of 'pins and needles'

30-year-old female referred with headaches
50-year-old female with angina and hypothyroidism
70-year-old man with asymptomatic hypertension.

General discussion questions:

Antibiotic prophylaxis of endocarditis
Autonomic neuropathy
Causes of late systolic murmurs
Diagnosis of brain stem death
Different types of herpetic infections
Diseases caused by animals
Epilepsy and driving
Haemoglobinuria
Harmful effects of alcohol
Histiocytosis X
Hypersensitivity: types and examples
Investigation of renal stones
Medical aspects of infertility
Medical causes of abdominal pain
Plasmapheresis
Renal tubular acidosis
Transfusion reactions.

Clinical pharmacology questions:

Drug interactions
Effects of opiate withdrawal
Indications for digoxin
Mechanism of action of acyclovir
Mode of action of different types of vasodilator drugs
Problems of drugs in the elderly
Properties of beta blocking drugs
Uses and side effects of: penicillamine, bromocriptine, captopril.

The management of medical emergencies:

Acute confusional states
Acute renal failure
Diabetic coma: ketotic/non-ketotic
Haematemesis/oesophageal varices
Hypercalcaemia
Hyperkalaemia

Hypertensive crisis
Hyperthermia/hypothermia
Meningitis, including cryptococcal
Pulmonary oedema (including use of Swan-Ganz catheter)
Status epilepticus
Thromboembolism in pregnancy
Unstable angina
A patient found 'collapsed' on the ward (cardiac arrest)
A young patient brought to casualty dyspnoeic and cyanosed (status asthmaticus).

Clinical physiology:

Effects of carbon dioxide retention
High altitude sickness
Physiological principles of the management of heart failure.
Respiratory function tests; significance of ventilation/perfusion abnormalities
The oxyhaemoglobin dissociation curve.

Pathology:

AIDS
Atypical mycobacteria
Classification of Hodgkin's disease
Effects of alcohol on the liver
Inappropriate ADH secretion
Menetrier's disease.

3 : THE LONG CASE

This is usually the least stressful part of the clinical. You have a full hour with a patient in which to take a history, carry out a physical examination and test the urine. There are three important rules to remember:

1. **Allocate your time carefully.**

   I suggest doing this as follows:

History	25 minutes
Examination plus urine testing	25 minutes
Planning of presentation, plus revision of difficult points in the history or examination	10 minutes

   You must keep a careful eye on the clock and be quite sure to leave enough time for the planning session. In fact, these last ten minutes are vitally important. It is your chance to edit and assemble your presentation. Furthermore, it is usually possible to predict the questions which you will be asked about the case and to have thought about your answers beforehand puts you at a great advantage.

2. **Establish a good rapport with your patient.**
   A common disaster is for the candidate to ask the patient at the beginning what is wrong with him. This is guaranteed to embarrass or annoy the patient, especially if he has been primed not to 'give the game away'. The candidate will then receive the classic reply, "That is for you to find out". Thus you *must* get the patient on your side. The best way to do this is simply to be polite, courteous and friendly. Introduce yourself and say where you are working. Take great care not to hurt the patient during the examination and check that he is warm enough and comfortable at all times. These, after all, are signs of a good doctor and will be recognised as such very quickly by most patients. In a way, the patient is your examiner for the first part of your meeting. If he decides that you are competent, courteous and not too full of yourself, you can be sure that he will do everything he can to ensure that you pass. It is not unheard of for sympathetic patients to point out difficult physical signs, e.g. "The consultant said that he could just feel my spleen under where your hand is now" or draw your attention to items of the history which you have missed: "You forgot to ask me whether I have worked with asbestos".

3. **Be thorough in your history and examination.**
   Long case patients often have complex medical histories but nevertheless, you should note everything initially and edit later.
   Take a complete drug history, including enquiry about side-effects. Do not forget a full social history where this is relevant. For example if the patient is wheelchair-bound you may be expected to know this in great detail. Smoking and drinking habits (past and present)should always be inquired about. Likewise, your physical examination should be absolutely complete, including testing of the urine. It is wise to note both the 4th and 5th Korotkoff sounds when recording the blood pressure.

Presenting the long case

You will now be led away from the patient to meet a pair of examiners. The session which follows usually opens in one of two ways; the first is the conventional approach, the request being made to "tell us about Mrs. Smith", at which point you must present your case just as you have prepared it. The alternative and less common way of opening is for the candidate to be asked directly about the patient's diagnosis or main problems. For example: "Before we go any further, what do you think is wrong with Mrs. Smith?" You should then, if possible, give a positive answer, such as, "I believe she has fibrosing alveolitis. This will be followed by a remark such as, "Why do you think that?" Whereupon, you should give the positive features in the history and examination.
This approach has been known to throw some candidates off their stride since they have to present their case in a different order.

You must make your presentation as concise and interesting as possible. This can only be achieved by making careful use of the planning period and as far as possible you must present the case without looking down at your notes. Always start conventionally with the patient's name, age and occupation and stick to the positive and important negative features of the history and examination. Long lists of negative findings are a sure way of enraging examiners. If, as is often the case, the patient has two or more separate complaints e.g. diabetes and asthma, it is sometimes a useful technique to describe the history of these separately. For example, "Mr. Brown is a fifty-four year old lorry driver. He has two main problems; diabetes and asthma. I will describe each of these in turn."

Remember that most physicians prefer drugs to be referred to by their approved names. Always mention the social history; considerable importance is often attached to this as it shows that you have considered the patient as a whole.

Again, with the physical examination you should describe only the positive and *important* negative findings. As I have said, you should be honest if you are completely ignorant on a subject about which you are asked. It is, however, bad technique to deliberately mention things of which you are not quite certain. There are times when it is much better to discuss difficult points only when specifically asked to do so.

To give an extreme example, you might have as your long case a 'neurological' patient with no obvious cardiovascular disorder. During the physical examination you are surprised at how easy it is to see the jugular venous pulse. You feel on balance, however, that this is a normal finding. This information should therefore be 'stored' for discussion if asked but should not be mentioned otherwise. The unwary candidate says in his presentation, "I found no definite abnormality in the cardiovascular system although I wondered whether the 'a' wave in the jugular venous pulse was possibly a little prominent." He has walked right into the lion's den! The chances are that he will be led back to the patient for a detailed analysis and discussion of the jugular venous pulse. Not only is this unpleasant enough on its own, but it is also time wasted as far as discussing things about which he does know is concerned. The rule is, therefore, to mention only those things which you are prepared to discuss.

Some candidates have an annoying habit of giving a list of the investigations which have been carried out on the patient. Although you should ask the patient about these, you should certainly not bring this into the presentation. Not only is this extremely boring but it will also give the examiners a feeling that you have in some way been cheating. In addition, it spoils the next part of the dialogue, which is generally "How would you investigate this patient?"

You will usually be given the results of any tests which you request and will be asked to comment on them: X-ray films are usually shown and your comments invited.

At this point you will probably be taken back to the patient to demonstrate the positive physical signs to the examiners. This resembles the short cases in some ways although it is generally much less stressful. I must emphasise again that if you have mentioned a physical sign, you will be asked to demonstrate it.

Just as in the short cases, you must show great care and consideration towards the patient as this is always being watched for.

Finally, you will probably return to the interview table and at this point you are likely to be asked how you would manage the patient. If you happen to know the patient's current management, it is wise not to disagree too wildly with this. The examination is not the place to argue about controversial subjects and in your own interests you should always bow to the greater experience of the examiners, even if you feel otherwise. In fact, you should be ready to learn during the examination and eagerness to do so is one way of creating the right impression.

If you have done well and there is still time, the discussion may turn to more specific questions about the pathology of the patient's condition or about the latest ideas as to its aetiology or management.

If the questions seem to be getting more difficult, you should not worry unduly; it usually means you have done well and that the examiners are now seeing how far you can go.

As in all the sections, be sure to thank the examiners at the end and to exit gracefully however you may be feeling.

4 : THE SHORT CASES

This is usually the most difficult part of the examination and I must repeat my advice to devote most of your preparation time to it. No amount of brilliance in the remainder of the examination will enable you to pass if you do not perform convincingly in this section.

Examining short cases is a skill which can only be mastered by careful planning and repeated rehearsal. You are expected to examine and answer questions on several patients in half an hour, six patients perhaps being an average number. The stress arises from the fact that you are being watched by two examiners throughout, both of whom know the correct diagnosis. Futhermore, you are not allowed to ask the patient any questions. You also have to be conscious of the time as it is to your advantage to see as many cases as possible in the half hour.

The examiners are trying to answer three questions about you:

1. Is your technique of examination thorough, systematic and effective?
2. Can you reliably detect abnormal physical signs and draw reasonable conclusions from them?
3. Are you professional in your manner and kind and considerate towards the patient?

There is, therefore, much more to the short cases than just getting the right diagnosis. In fact, occasional mistakes, if of a minor nature, maybe forgiven if your overall performance and approach are good. For example a candidate who correctly elicits the signs of upper lobe pulmonary fibrosis but, in his anxious state, fails to notice a small scar overlying this site, might still pass if his performance in the other cases were well above average. In this regard, first impressions are most important. If you perform well in your first short case, the examiners will tend to relax and take a more kindly view of subsequent errors. It is important, therefore, to practice getting straight into the cases; it is not enough to warm up on the first case.

Planning your examination technique is important in the short cases and I will discuss this shortly. However, the essence of preparation boils down to one thing: *you must make yourself examine patients repeatedly in front of an observer.* Here, to team up with a like-minded candidate, as suggested in Chapter 1 is most useful. You should take it in turns to play the examiner: a most valuable exercise in itself as it gives insight into the sorts of questions that are likely to be asked. Avoid the temptation to spend most of your preparation time in the library: this is the best way to fail.

Each short case consists of two parts: the examination and the presentation of findings:

Examination technique

The inexperienced candidate often makes the mistake of diving straight into the physical examination. The preliminaries need not take more than half a minute but are most important in creating a good impression. In each case you will be taken to the patient and requested to perform a specific examination; for example, "Examine this man's cardiovascular system". Be most careful to follow the examiners' instructions. For example, if asked to examine the abdomen (rather than the abdominal system), do just that; you can look at the hands, etc. afterwards if necessary. Similarly, if asked to "Examine the precordium" (a frequent request), do not start by feeling the pulse.

Whatever the request, you should start by shaking hands with, and introducing yourself to, the patient and by asking him whether he minds if you examine him. You should then, again with the patient's permission, make sure that the patient is undressed adequately to allow a complete examination of the system specified. If you omit to do this, not only will the examiners lose confidence in you from the beginning, but you will also greatly reduce your chances of detecting abnormal physical signs. Adequate exposure can reveal all sorts of hidden clues: biopsy scars in the groin and neck are classic examples of this, as are thyroidectomy scars. Indeed, it is not unheard of for your approach to be tested in this way. For example, you may be asked to examine the chest in an elderly lady who has had a stroke. The important point, for which the examiners are looking, is not to compromise. You must arrange the patient in the correct position with the chest exposed, despite all the practical difficulties involved in a case such as this. Be absolutely stringent about this; short cuts can lead to your downfall.

At this point the unprepared usually forget one important act: *observation*. Observing the patient need not take more than a few seconds but will impress the examiners and will quite often give you the diagnosis. Just as in the driving test you must be sure to be seen checking the rear view mirror, in the Membership examination you must be certain that the examiners see you stand back and observe the patient, the end of the bed being a traditional vantage point. Do not forget to look for clues by the patient's bed, such as a bottle of diabetic orange juice or a salbutamol inhaler.

All the steps of the examination should be clear to the onlookers and follow on quickly and smoothly from one another. Repeated practice is the only way to achieve this and those who have done this can be recognised within seconds of starting their examination of a patient.

When you have finished examining each case, be sure to thank the patient and to help him back on with his clothes.

Occasionally, an examiner will ask you to give a running commentary during your examination. You should practise doing this on a few occasions. Even more off-putting is being stopped in mid-examination and asked to "Present your findings up to now." Again, to practise this with your 'team-mate' can be helpful.

Presenting your findings

As soon as you straighten up from examining the patient you will be asked "What did you find?"

There are two ways of presenting your findings.

1. **If you are sure of the diagnosis** you should state this, followed by your reasons. An example would be "This patient has Parkinson's disease, as shown by a coarse pill-rolling tremor of the hands at rest, cogwheel rigidity of the arms, . . . " etc.

   This method of presentation has many advantages; not only does it make you sound confident, but it also gives you much more control over what you include and what you omit from your presentation. As mentioned in the discussion on the long case, there are times when it is better not to mention signs about which you are not sure; to some extent, everything you say can be used in evidence against you!

2. **If you are not sure of the diagnosis** you should go through your findings methodically and at the end give a probable diagnosis or differential diagnosis. Do not lose your nerve or apologise for not knowing the diagnosis; often this is not actually expected of you. Many cases are chosen to test your clinical approach rather than your ability to 'spot the diagnosis'. There are times when to be too definite can stand against you. For example, you might be shown a patient with jaundice and a firm enlarged liver. It would be wrong to say "This patient has hepatic secondaries." This should certainly enter into your

differential, but to give it as a firm diagnosis would indicate lack of clinical experience.

Very occasionally, after you have examined the case, you will be allowed to "Ask the patient a few questions". Another short case variant is to be asked to examine a specific region "and anything else you feel is relevant". This is a good way of testing your knowledge of clinical associations. If you have prepared properly, your mind should already be thinking of these associations in any case, as I will now describe.

Mastering the case

The membership will always be a competitive examination, with candidates before and after you being tested on the same patients. To impress your examiners you should consider how to take your examination one step further after you have reached a diagnosis. Planning this aspect is one of the most stimulating and enjoyable parts of preparing for the Membership.

To illustrate this, let us take the following example. You are led to a patient with obvious rheumatoid arthritis and asked to examine the hands (in fact, an extremely common short case). The immediate reaction is to breathe a sigh of relief because at last you will be able to give a confident diagnosis. Unfortunately, so could a first year medical student! It is these cases which call for the slickest performance and the ability to examine the case in greater depth than that of the average candidate. In the case of rheumatoid hands, for example, you would make a good impression, after a thorough examination of the various features of the disease, by performing some simple bedside tests of function, such as doing up buttons, or writing. This indicates a practical approach to the patient's disability; something which cannot be learned from books and which is likely to go down very well with the examiners, especially if they have just seen several half-hearted examinations of the same patient's hands by less well prepared candidates.

Similarly, having diagnosed mitral stenosis you should look for and comment on the presence or absence of complications of the condition rather than letting the examiners drag this information out of you.

Further examples of this approach are mentioned in the notes on popular short cases.

Planning your revision

As I have said already, the only way to master the technique of handling short cases is to practise them repeatedly in front of someone in the wards. However, there is a lot to be gained by planning out on paper your method of tackling different short case situations, especially those which tend to crop up regularly.

It is worthwhile making lists of the signs which accompany the various conditions which occur as short cases. There are many books available to help you do this but be sure to make your *own* lists because you will remember much better what you have written down yourself.

This method of preparation has one important limitation: although some short cases are immediately diagnosable 'from the end of the bed', on many occasions this is not so, and the diagnosis only becomes clear at the end of the examination, if at all! On those lucky occasions when the diagnosis *is* obvious it certainly helps to be able to switch into a prepared routine of examination as, for example, with rheumatoid arthritis or Parkinson's disease. For the other occasions, it is vital to be absolutely systematic about your method of examination. You must prepare and rehearse a method of thoroughly examining each system of the body. Your normal methods will probably need to be adjusted and 'race-tuned' for the rigours of the short cases. Not only must your technique be smooth and well-polished, but you must incorporate certain safety checks, such as feeling both radial pulses to avoid being caught out by an absent radial.

To help you with this aspect of your preparation I have compiled some schemes of suggested examination technique which are given in the next chapter.

5 : SCHEMES OF EXAMINATION TECHNIQU

No method of examination is *correct* and you should modify these methods so that they feel natural to you in practice and can be performed smoothly and automatically even when under stress.

These schemes of examination technique are followed by a selection of popular short cases.

"Examine the cardiovascular system"

Action	*Notes*
Introduce yourself and ask permission to examine the patient.	
Position patient with top half undressed at 45 degrees to horizontal.	
Stand at end of bed and observe.	*? malar flush* *? tachypnoeic* *? scars (e.g. sternotomy)* *? marfanoid appearance*
Examine radial pulse (see p.36).	*rate; rhythm*
Check other radial pulse simultaneously.	*? absent radial*
In younger patients, check for radiofemoral delay. Lift arm and feel for 'radial knock'.	
Glance at antecubital fossa for catheter scars.	
Look at eye.	*? anaemic* *?Argyll-Robertson pupil*
Look at tongue.	*? central cyanosis*
Palpate carotid pulse.	*? abnormal character*
Examine jugular venous pulse (height from sternal angle and wave form see p.38)	

Examine apex for position and character of beat.	*check for valvotomy scars at this point*
Feel for heaves and thrills at apex, and to left and right of sternum.	
Listen at apex with bell.	*Time the heart sounds by palpating the patient's right carotid pulse simultaneously*
Repeat auscultation at apex with patient in left lateral position.	*? mid-diastolic* *? mid-diastolic murmur*
Reposition patient comfortably.	
Listen with diaphragm at: a) apex b) below sternum c) 2nd right intercostal space d) left sternal edge.	
Ask patient to sit forward and listen again with diaphragm at c) and d) with breath held in expiration.	*? early diastolic murmur*
Listen at lung bases.	
Inspect for sacral oedema.	
Inspect for ankle oedema.	
Ask examiner whether he wishes you to examine the peripheral pulses or to measure the blood pressure.	

"Examine the respiratory system"

Action	*Notes*
Introduce yourself and ask permission to examine the patient.	
Position patient comfortably in upright sitting position with chest fully undressed.	
Check bedside locker for sputum pot and inspect this if present.	
Look quickly at hands for clubbing or peripheral cyanosis.	
Feel radial pulse and count respiratory rate.	*? rapid, bounding pulse of CO_2 retention, check for flapping tremor if you suspect this.*
Glance at pupils and conjunctivae.	*? Horner's syndrome* *? anaemic/polycythaemic*
Look at tongue.	*? central cyanosis*
Stand at end of bed and observe while patient breathes in.	*? scars; deformities* *? asymmetrical expansion*
Further assess expansion anteriorly by palpation.	
Palpate trachea and apex beat.	
Percuss chest anteriorly.	*Do not forget to percuss over the clavicles*
Palpate for tactile fremitus.	
Auscultate anteriorly, including over the apices.	*if crepitations are heard ask the patient*

Auscultate for vocal resonance anteriorly.

to cough, then repeat auscultation

Ask patient to sit forward.

Assess expansion posteriorly by palpation.

Percuss posteriorly, including the axillae.

Palpate for tactile fremitus.

Auscultate posteriorly, including axillae.

When consolidation is suspected, check for additional signs such as increased vocal resonance, whispering pectoriloquy and aegophony

Auscultate for vocal resonance posteriorly.

Palpate for cervical, supraclavicular and axillary lymphadenopathy.

"Examine the abdominal system"

Action	*Notes*
Introduce yourself and ask permission to examine the patient.	
Position patient lying flat on the bed with one pillow. Expose abdomen completely, including inguinal regions but not genitalia.	
Look quickly at hands for clubbing, leuconychia, Dupuytren's contracture, liver palms, splinter haemorrhages, spider naevi.	*All these observations should be carried out very quickly as it is usually the abdomen which contains the major abnormality*
Glance at sclerae for jaundice,	

conjunctivae for anaemia.

Look for spider naevi on the face and chest.

Inspect the tongue.

Palpate cervical and supraclavicular lymph nodes.

Stand at end of bed and observe the abdomen while the patient takes a deep breath.

Kneel on the floor or sit on a chair so that you are relaxed and palpate the abdomen.

with a high bed this may not be practical

First do a 'scout' palpation for massses or organomegaly. Initially palpate lightly, asking the patient to let you know if there is any tenderness.

NB Large masses, spleens or livers are often visible on inspection. This makes the rest of the examination much easier

Then palpate again more deeply.

If you find a mass, determine its characteristics at this stage.

Palpate groin for glands. Check hernial orifices.

Palpate for the liver and percuss out its upper and lower borders.

If liver is enlarged auscultate over it for a bruit

Palpate for a spleen. In difficult cases ask the patient to roll onto his right side.

Palpate for renal enlargement.

Percuss for ascites and test for shifting dullness, if this is suspected.

Auscultate abdomen for bruits (especially on either side of umbilicus for renal artery stenosis) and bowel sounds

Tell the examiners that you would normally both examine the genitalia and perform a rectal examination.

Causes of abdominal bruits:
Systolic bruit over liver: hepatoma, alcoholic hepatitis (occasionally)

Venous hum in region of umbilicus or xiphoid in portal hypertension due to collateral flow *(see Sherlock p.138)*

Bruits of renal artery Stenosis - lateral to umbilicus or in loins

"Examine the cranial nerves"

Note: this examination is one in which the candidate who has prepared carefully can readily be distinguished from those who have not.

Practice the 'routine' repeatedly, using this or your own scheme. You should be able to get through it in three or four minutes.

Introduce yourself and ask permission to examine the patient.

I	Ask "Has there been any change in your sense of smell recently?"
II	Quickly check visual acuity using your pocket reading chart. If the patient wears glasses, he should put them on. Test visual fields with white hat pin. Look for ptosis. Observe pupils and test reaction to light and accommodation. Examine the fundi.
III , IV VI	Test eye movements and observe for nystagmus.
V	Test facial sensation briefly (use cotton wool on both sides). Test corneal reflexes. Test pterygoids "Open your mouth and don't let me close it".

Test masseters "Clench your teeth". Palpate muscles simultaneously.
Test jaw jerk.

VII Test facial muscles:

"Smile"
"Show me your teeth"
"Blow your cheeks out like this"
"Raise your eyebrows like this"
"Screw your eyes up tightly and don't let me open them".

VIII Test hearing with a watch: (A watch on a chain is useful for this: digital watches are not.)

"Do you hear my watch ticking? Tell me when the sound disappears.

Perform Rinne's and Weber's tests (see below).

X, IX Observe uvula. "Open your mouth and say aah".

XI Test sternocleidomastoids: "Push your chin against my hand". Palpate muscle simultaneously.

Test trapezii: "Shrug your shoulders. Push down simultaneously.

XII Look for wasting, fasciculation of the non-protruded tongue.

Look for deviation and weakness: "Push your tongue out straight.
Now move it from side to side.

Weber's and Rinne's Tests

	CONDUCTIVE DEAFNESS	SENSINEURAL DEAFNESS
Rinne	BC > AC (negative Rinne) IN DEAF EAR	AC > BC BOTH EARS*
Weber	SOUND REFERRED TO DEAF EAR	SOUND REFERRED TO BETTER EAR

*False negative Rinne may occur in severe sensineural deafness: bone conducted sound heard in good ear.

BC=bone condition AC=air condition

"Examine the patients upper limbs"

Action	*Notes*
1. Inspect hands:	
skin	
nails	
joints (? arthropathy see p.28)	
muscles (? wasting see p.91 ? tremor see p.95)	
2. Inspect arms: skin (especially elbows). Lesions at the elbow common in the short cases include:	

Psoriatic plaques
Rheumatoid nodules
Xanthomata (see p.117)
Gouty tophi (may involve olecranon bursa)
Lesions of Pseudoxanthomata Elasticum (see p.82)
Subcutaneous calcification

Muscles

3. **Check pulses bilaterally**

4. **Palpate for axillary lymph nodes**

If the above are negative, proceed to neurological examination.

"Carry out a neurological examination of this patients upper limbs"

Introduce yourself and ask the patient's permission to examine his arms. Make sure that the arms are adequately exposed. Look for (and be seen looking for) wasting, fasciculation and scars.

1. **Assess tone:**

"Let your arm and hand go loose and let me move them for you." (Start at the wrist and move upwards.)

2. **Test power:**

Start by asking the patient to hold his arms outstretched and then to close his eyes.
Observe for weakness, parietal drift, or oscillations (*see J.Patten p. 72*)

Now proceed rapidly through the muscle groups, starting proximally (as proximal weakness is a common short case):

Action	*Notes*
"I'm going to test the strength of some of your muscles."	
"Hold your arms out to your sides, like this . . . Now keep them up and don't let me stop you."	*shoulder abduction: Deltoids C5*
"Now push them in towards you and don't let me stop you."	*shoulder adduction: Pectorals C6, 7, 8*
"Pull your arms up towards you and don't let me stop you."	*arm flexion: Biceps C5*
"Now push me away."	*arm extension: Triceps C7*
"Clench your fists and bend your wrists up towards you. Don't let me stop you."	*wrist flexors: C7*
"Now push the other way."	*wrist extensors: C7*
"Grip my fingers tightly (use two of your fingers)."	*long and short flexors: C8, T1*
"Put your hand down flat, like this (palm upwards) . . ., and point your thumb towards your nose. Now keep it there and don't let me push it down."	*thumb abduction: Abductor pollucis brevis; median nerve C8, T1*
"Spread your fingers wide apart and don't let me push them together."	*finger abduction: Dorsal interossei; ulnar nerve T1*
"Now hold this piece of card between your fingers and don't let me pull it away."	*finger adduction Palmar interossei; ulnar nerve T1*

Describe any weakness in terms of the Medical Research Council scale:

Grade		
Grade	0	No movement
	1	Flicker of movement on voluntary contraction
	2	Movement present but not against gravity
	3	Movement against gravity but not against resistance
	4	Movement against resistance but not full strength
	5	Full strength.

3. **Test reflexes**

Biceps	C5/6	
Supinator	C5/6	If absent, test with reinforcement
Triceps	C7	

4. **Test sensation** (NB: You must be familiar with the anatomical sites of the different dermatomes.)

A **Pinprick** (Use each end of the hat pin.)

First demonstrate the stimuli to the patient by testing on the sternum: "This is sharp . . . and this is blunt . . . Now I 'm going to test the sensation in your arms and I want you to close your eyes and say "Sharp" if it feels sharp, and "Blunt" if it feels blunt.
Test over each dermatome of each arm quickly.
If sensation to pinprick is impaired, test temperature sensation using tuning fork (cold) and your hand (warm).

B **Light touch**

"I want you to say 'Yes' if you feel me touch you with this piece of cotton wool." (NB Do not stroke the skin as this tests tickle, which travels in the spinothalamic tract.)

C **Joint position sense**

Start with the distal interphalangeal joint of one finger. "I'm going to move your finger up and down; this is up (move finger up) . . ., and this is down (move finger down) . . . Now close your eyes and tell me whether I am moving your finger up or down." If the patient cannot do this move to more proximal joints progressively.

D **Vibration sense**

Make the fork vibrate silently (practice this):
"Do you feel this vibrating." (Test on sternum.)
"Can you feel it vibrating now?" (Test on distal interphalangeal joint of one finger.)

If patient cannot feel the vibration, move progressively to more proximal joints.

5. **Test coordination**

"Touch my finger with your index finger. Now touch your nose." (Move patient's hand for him once if he has difficulty in understanding what is required.) "Now do the same as quickly as possible and keep going."

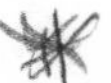

Examination of arthritic hands

Ask the patient's permission to examine his hands and then observe carefully for: *joint swelling* and *deformities.* The pattern of joint involvement is all-important and should be carefully noted.

Look for characteristic rheumatoid deformities:

swan-neck
boutonnière
Z-deformity of thumb
ulnar deviation of fingers
dorsal subluxation of ulna at carpal joint.

Ask the patient whether his hands are painful before touching them. Then pick up the hands and examine:

nails for thimble-pitting or nail fold infarcts
clubbing as in hypertrophic pulmonary osteoarthropathy (NB wrists)
temperature over joints

Check for:

rheumatoid nodules
Heberden's or Bouchard's nodes

gouty tophi
synovial effusions in tendon sheaths.

Observe and palpate for wasting of the small muscles of the hand. Note whether the skin is atrophic (often secondary to steroid therapy).

Turn the hand over so that the palm faces upwards and observe for palmar erythema (see p.70).

Look quickly at the elbows for psoriatic plaques or rheumatoid nodules and if you suspect gout, look at the helices of the ears for tophi.

Test the grip and pincer movements and quickly test for evidence of median or ulnar nerve compression. (Test abductor pollucis brevis and interossei and compare sensation with pinprick over index and little fingers.)

Get the patient to perform a simple test of hand function, such as undoing a button, or writing.

"Examine this patient's lower limbs"

Here again, you should list the various abnormalities which you might observe at each step of the examination.

Action	*Notes*
Observe:	
Skin NB ulcers, see p.123 Do not forget soles of feet and between toes Lesions on shins, see p.122	
Joints/bones NB swollen knee joint, see p.133 Paget's disease, see p.138	
Muscles	
Calves/ankles (Look carefully for oedema, see p.124)	

Palpate peripheral pulses and inguinal nodes. Auscultate over femoral arteries.

If the above are negative, proceed to neurological examination.

"Carry out a neurological examination of this patient's lower limbs"

Introduce yourself and ask permission to examine the patient. Ensure that the legs are fully exposed but also make sure that the patient remains 'decent'. Observe for wasting and fasciculation.

1. **Assess tone:**

   "Let your leg go loose and let me move it for you" Use more than one method: roll the leg from the knee, then with a hand behind the knee, flex the leg and feel for any 'catch'. Then passively flex the leg at the knee and hip joints. If tone is increased, test for knee and ankle clonus.

2 **Test power** (start proximally):

"I'm going to test the strength of some of the muscles in your legs. Keep your leg straight and lift it up into the air. Now keep it up and don't let me stop you."	*hip flexion:* *Iliopsoas L1,2*
"Now push your leg down into the bed and don't let me stop you."	*hip extension:* *Glutei L4,5*
"Push out against my hand."	*hip abduction* *Glutei L4,5*
"Push in against my hand."	*hip adduction:* *Adductor group L2.3.4*

Instruction	Movement and muscle
"Bend your knee and pull your heel up towards you: don't let me stop you." (Hold ankle.)	*knee flexion:* *Hamstrings L5,S1*
"Now straighten your knee out."	*knee extention:* *Quadriceps L3,4*
"Pull your foot up to you and don't let me stop you."	*ankle dorsiflexion:* *Tibialis anterior and long extensors L4,5*
"Push your foot down against my hand."	*ankle plantar flexion:* *Gastrocnemius S1*
"Push your foot out against my hand."	*eversion of foot:* *Peronei S1*
"Push your foot in against my hand."	*inversion of foot* *Tibiais anterior and posterior L4*

Any weakness should be described in terms of the Medical Research Council scale.

3. **Test reflexes:**

   Knee L4
   Ankle S1 If absent, test with reinforcement.

4. **Test plantar responses:** use an 'orange stick' (*see Patten p.141*).

5. **Test sensation:**

   Pin-prick, light touch, vibration sense and joint position sense as described for the upper limbs. When testing joint position sense remember to hold the lateral aspect of the big toe *(see Patten p.74)*.

6. **Test coordination:**

   Use the heel-shin test.

7. **Perform Romberg's test**

Tell the examiners that you would like to examine the patient's gait.

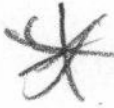

"Examine the patient's neck (or thyroid gland)"

Ask permission to examine the patient and ensure that the neck is adequately exposed.

Observe:

1. Is the jugular venous pressure elevated? (see p.38)
2. Are there any scars?
3. Are there any enlarged lymph glands visible? If so, proceed to examine the neck glands thoroughly (see lymphadenopathy p.33)
4. Is there an obvious goitre? (the commonest example of this short case)

If there is an obvious goitre:

Arrange the patient comfortably in a chair.
Give the patient a glass of water, there is usually one conveniently nearby! Inspect and palpate the gland from the front.
Stand behind the patient and palpate the gland, one lobe at a time. The patient should be asked to swallow some water, at appropriate intervals.

You should be assessing:

a) size
b) texture: smooth or nodular; solitary or multiple nodules.
c) mobility
d) tenderness.

Palpate the cervical lymph glands.

Check for tracheal displacement.
Percuss for retrosternal extension.
If there is a thyroidectomy scar, test for Chvostek's sign.
Auscultate over the gland for bruits.

Now perform simple tests of thyroid function:

Observe for myxoedematous facies.
Feel pulse (check rate, rhythm and volume).
Feel palms (? sweaty). Look for palmar erythema.
Ask patient to hold hands outstretched. Look for postural tremor.
Inspect for acropachy.
Test supinator jerks (observe relaxation phase).
Test for thyroid eye disease. Look for exophthalmos; test for opthalmoplegia (use white hat pin) and lid lag.
If you suspect hyperthyroidism, test for proximal myopathy by testing shoulder abduction.
Observe shins: ? pretibial myxoedema.
Tell the examiner that you would like to ask the patient if he has any difficulty in breathing or swallowing.

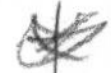

Lymphadenopathy

Enlarged cervical lymph glands are common as a short case. Look for a scar from lymph node biopsy and for radiotherapy markings.

Now examine methodically the deep cervical, tonsillar, submandibular, submental, occipital, posterior triangle and supraclavicular nodes.

Always look in the mouth for

a) pharyngitis and palatal petechiae (seen in infectious mononucleosis)
b) tonsillar infiltration, (sometimes seen in chronic lymphocytic leukaemia)
c) primary malignancies.

If allowed, proceed to examine for generalised lymphadenopathy (palpate axillary, epitrochlear and inguinal nodes) and for enlargement of the liver and spleen. Comment on the desirability of clinical and radiological examination of the chest (TB or carcinoma).

When asked the differential diagnosis, consider common causes first:

Localised cervical lymphadenopathy.

* Infection: tonsillitis, tuberculosis.
* Lymphoma, especially Hodgkin's.
* Secondary carcinoma. Remember nasopharyngeal carcinoma which may need to be excluded by ENT examination.

N.B. Troisier's sign (Virchow's nodes): enlargement of left supraclavicular nodes suggestive of carcinoma of the stomach.

Generalised lymphadenopathy

Common causes are:

* lymphomas
* chronic lymphocytic leukaemia
* infections: acute: infectious mononucleosis, cytomegalovirus, toxoplasmosis
  chronic: tuberculosis, brucellosis, syphilis (now rare).

Other causes worth remembering are phenytoin and AIDS.

Always include in your differential diagnosis both systemic lupus erythematosus (look for butterfly rash) and sarcoidosis (look for skin lesions, e.g. erythema nodosum).

"Examine this man's eyes"

1. **Observe for presence of:**

   exophthalmos
   ptosis
   squint
   xanthelasmata
   arcus
   corneal calcification
   blue sclerae
   Kayser-Fleischer rings
   thyroidectomy scar (always check for this as it gives a strong clue as to the presence of thyroid eye disease).

2. **Test visual acuity** in both eyes using pocket reading chart.

   If patient wears glasses these should be worn to correct for refractive errors.

3. **Test eye movements** (ask patient to follow white hat pin with his eyes and to report any double vision).

   Observe at the same time for nystagmus, both horizontal and vertical. Diplopia and nystagmus are such common short cases that I recommend testing for them at this early stage.

4. **Test visual fields**

   Quickly check for visual inattention using fingers. Then test visual fields in each eye using white hat pin.

5. **Examine pupils**

   Observe for dilatation, constriction or irregularity.
   Test reactions to light and accommodation. (Beware the glass eye which reacts to neither!)

6. **Examine the fundi** checking first for the red reflex.

   Ask the examiner whether he wishes you to examine the corneal reflex.

6 : POPULAR SHORT CASES

These lists of popular short cases are in no way intended to be comprehensive and you should add other possible short cases which you think of or hear of from recent candidates.

Below each case are notes on problems, points to remember or examination hints. A space is provided in which you should make your own notes on signs and associations of the various conditions.

CARDIOVASCULAR SHORT CASES

You are almost certain to be given at least one cardiac case to diagnose. This is one area in which you can improve greatly and quickly with practice and you must repeatedly examine cardiac cases until you are confident in your ability to recognise the common heart valve lesions.

Remember that since many cardiac lesions can be suspected or diagnosed before auscultation, you must concentrate carefully on all the steps prior to this.

Revise the signs which you would expect to find in each of the following cases using the space provided to make your own notes.

"Examine this patient's pulse"

First check the rate and rhythm at the radial pulse (wear a watch with a second hand.). Revise the common causes of sinus tachycardia, sinus bradycardia (NB drugs e.g. beta-blockers), atrial fibrillation and complete heart block.

If you suspect complete heart block, look for cannon waves in the jugular venous pulse as well as regular 'a' waves occurring more rapidly than the ventricular rate, and variability of the intensity of the first heart sound: remember that a basal systolic ejection murmur is usually present due to increased stroke volume.

In atrial fibrillation 'a' waves will be absent; again the first heart sound varies in intensity. Assess the rate both at the radial pulse and apex and comment on the pulse deficit.

Next *always* palpate both radial pulses simultaneously. Absent radial pulse occurs as a short case: common causes include congenital, trauma or surgery (e.g. cardiac catheter, Blalock shunt), systemic embolisation (e.g. mitral stenosis; patient usually in atrial fibrillation).

Elevate the arm and feel for 'knock' of a collapsing pulse against your palm.

Always palpate for radiofemoral delay to avoid missing aortic coarctation.

Always palpate a large artery, e.g. the carotid, to assess the volume and character of the pulse. Remember that the carotids may be *visible* in aortic regurgitation (Corrigan's sign see p.43).

Remember to listen over the carotid and femoral arteries for bruits.

Common cases include:

1. Collapsing pulse (steep upstroke and downstroke). Seen not only in aortic regurgitation but also in presence of large a-v fistulae (occcuring on rare occasions in Paget's disease) and patent ductus arteriosus. A large volume (but not collapsing) pulse also occurs in high output states e.g. anaemia, thyrotoxicosis, beri-beri.

2. Slow rising, plateau or anacrotic pulse of aortic stenosis.

3. Bisferiens pulse of combined aortic stenosis and regurgitation.

4. Occasionally pulsus alternans or paradoxus.

Notes

Jugular Venous Pulse

Always be meticulous in positioning the patient at 45 degrees to the horizontal.

If internal jugular venous pulse is not visible immediately:

1. Check for a low level by

   a) pressing on the liver (ask first if this is tender): remember that hepatojugular reflux may have no patho-physiological significance.

   b) lying patient more horizontally.

2. Check for a very high pressure, look at the ear lobes (these may move with cardiac cycle) and sit the patient vertical.

Measure the vertical height of jugular venous pulse above the sternal angle; in normal individuals this is not more than 2-4cm. If the pressure is very high the hand veins may be used as a manometer, as they collapse when the hand is held at the appropriate height above the right atrium.

Identify the two main waves by simultaneously palpating the opposite carotid artery ('a' wave just prior to systole; 'v' wave during systole).

Remember that there is no 'a' wave in atrial fibrillation.

The most likely short cases are:

1. Large 'v' waves (tricuspid regurgitation): palpate for systolic impulse in liver and auscultate for murmur (see p.46).

2. Large 'a' waves: pulmonary stenosis, pulmonary hypertension or tricuspid stenosis: palpate and auscultate over pulmonary area.

3. Cannon waves:

   Irregular: complete heart block, multiple extrasystoles,
   Regular: 2:1 atrio-ventricular block.
   nodal rhythm (usually)

A steep y descent occurs with any cause of raised jugular venous pressure, especially constrictive pericarditis (NB Kussmaul's sign, rise in jugular venous pressure on inspiration).

Superior vena caval obstruction (p. 62) causes nonpulsatile elevation of the jugular venous pressure, not affected by pressure on the neck or abdomen.

Finally in any case of raised jugular venous pressure check for other signs of congestive cardiac failure: ankle and sacral oedema, tender hepatomegaly, basal crackles or pleural effusions.

Notes

Mitral stenosis

This is an extremely common short case in which you can excel if you are well prepared. Revise the signs of the condition and make notes in the space provided. Remember to exercise the patient to bring out the diastolic murmur if you are suspicious or unsure of it.

As well as making the diagnosis you should always comment on the severity of the stenosis (mild, moderate or severe).

Indicators of severity are:

1. Distance from the second heart sound to the opening snap (this reflects left atrial pressure).

2. Duration of the diastolic murmur.

A guide to severity on auscultation is:

a) Mild stenosis: diastolic murmur occupies half diastole. opening snap is late (>100 msecs after A_2).

b) Moderate stenosis: diastolic murmur almost fills diastole. opening snap about 80 msecs after A_2.

c) Severe stenosis: diastolic murmur extends throughout diastole. early opening snap (<60 msecs after A_2).

Note: None but the very experienced can put a time in milliseconds to the distance between A_2 and opening snap and unless you are very confident about this, it would be unwise to do so).

If possible, you should comment on the pliability of the mitral valve.

Remember that if the valve becomes rigid or calcified, the first sound becomes less loud and the opening snap may disappear.

You should also mention the presence or absence of complications:

1 Atrial fibrillation.

2. Pulmonary hypertension:

   a) Palpable and loud P_2
   b) Large 'a' waves in the jugular venous pulse (remember that these disappear if the patient is in atrial fibrillation).
   c) Left parasternal heave due to associated right ventricular hypertrophy.

d) In severe cases there may be an early diastolic murmur at the left sternal edge due to pulmonary regurgitation (Graham Steell murmur).

e) Pulmonary ejection click due to dilated pulmonary artery.

3. Right ventricular failure (N.B. the diastolic murmur may become soft or inaudible).

4. Tricuspid regurgitation (common in advanced stenosis, see p.46).

It is better to comment spontaneously on the severity of stenosis, pliability of the valve and presence of complications than to have this information dragged out of you.

Patients with more than one valvular lesion often appear in the Membership. A particularly common example is aortic regurgitation with mitral stenosis. Here one may be faced with the possibility that an apical mid-diastolic murmur is an Austin-Flint murmur. This sounds exactly like that of mitral stenosis and may even have presystolic accentuation. The first heart sound may sometimes be accentuated and is of no help in differentiation. The opening snap is however of help, being absent in the case of an Austin-Flint murmur. Its presence, therefore, confirms mitral stenosis (although its absence does not exclude this diagnosis as it may disappear when the valve is rigid).

The presence of atrial fibrillation also favours the existence of mitral stenosis. In practice, echocardiography is valuable in distinguishing these two causes of mid-diastolic murmurs.

Notes

Mitral regurgitation/mixed mitral valve disease

Revise the causes of this common short case. Remember that in mitral *regurgitation* (but not stenosis) the apex beat may be displaced downwards and outwards and be thrusting in character; a third heart sound is common (*not* a feature of stenosis) and there may be a soft mid-diastolic murmur due to rapid left ventricular filling.

Mixed mitral valve disease is also common: the problem many candidates have is to decide which is the dominant lesion. The following is a guide to features which, if present, aid in this decision:

Dominant mitral regurgitation:

* Apex beat displaced and thrusting.
* Third sound rather than opening snap.

Dominant mitral stenosis:

* 'Tapping apex' but not displaced.
* Loud dominant mid-diastolic murmur.
* Loud first heart sound.
* Opening snap rather than third sound.
* Evidence of severe pulmonary hypertension.

A word of warning: never forget to look carefully for a mitral valvotomy scar during your cardiac examination. Remember that after valvotomy the loud first sound and opening snap remain, but diastolic murmurs are shortened or abolished. Some patients, however, develop a degree of mitral regurgitation, and re-stenosis may occur, so that these patients may have the signs of mixed mitral valve disease.

Notes

Aortic regurgitation

An extremely common short case. Usually the collapsing pulse should make you suspect the diagnosis at the beginning of your examination; this is the value of *routinely* feeling for a radial 'knock' against your palm with the patient's arm held vertically upwards.

Examine the apex carefully for displacement and thrusting character.

The early diastolic murmur is sometimes difficult to hear: *always* sit the patient forward with the breath held in expiration and listen at the left sternal edge with the diaphragm.

Remember that an ejection systolic murmur is a common finding and does not necessarily imply the presence of aortic stenosis (see mixed aortic valve disease p45). The Austin Flint murmur should be listened for (see mitral stenosis, p.39). Listen at the lung bases for evidence of left ventricular failure. *Always* tell the examiners that you would like to check the blood pressure.

Do not start to search for additional signs until you have completed the main cardiac examination. If you have time, you may then look very quickly for

* visible carotid pulsation (Corrigan's sign)
* head bobbing (de Musset's sign)
* capillary pulsation of nail beds (Quincke's sign).

You can ask the examiner if you may listen over the femoral arteries for:

a) pistol shot sounds synchronous with the pulse (Traube's sign).
b) to and fro murmur on light compression with diaphragm, the diastolic component of which is diagnostic of aortic regurgitation (Duroziez's sign).

Glance for evidence of rare causes, e.g. Marfan's syndrome, syphilis (Argyll-Robertson pupil), ankylosing spondylitis, rheumatoid arthritis.

Notes

Aortic stenosis

You must be able to recognise the slow rising pulse of this condition (often with an early notch on the upstroke); it should alert you to its existence at the very beginning of the examination. A palpable thrill may be present in the carotids. Remember that the apex tends to be sustained and heaving but is not usually displaced (except in very severe disease when the left ventricle has dilated); there may be an additional palpable presystolic apical impulse due to atrial systole.

Palpate carefully for a systolic thrill in the second right intercostal space.

Listen carefully to the second heart sound: it may be soft if the valve is heavily calcified; paradoxical splitting may occur. There may be a *fourth sound*, and an *ejection click* (in valvar stenosis), the latter disappearing if the valve becomes heavily calcified. The murmur is often heard *all over the precordium* (unlike that of mitral regurgitation); listen for radiation to the carotids. Remember that occasionally the murmur is heard maximally at the left sternal edge or apex. A degree of aortic regurgitation often coexists so always listen carefully at the left sternal edge for a diastolic murmur in the usual way. Look also for mitral valve disease (it often coexists if the stenosis is rheumatic in origin; atrial fibrillation may give a clue to this possibility).

Always ask if you may take the patient's blood pressure (check for narrow pulse pressure) but note that a normal or even high pulse pressure or systolic pressure does not exclude the diagnosis. Note also that the murmur may soften in the presence of left ventricular failure. The condition must be distinguished from HOCM (see p.48) and aortic sclerosis. In the latter condition the pulse is normal in character, as is the apex beat and the second sound; there is no ejection click or systolic thrill and the murmur does not generally radiate to the carotid arteries. However, with the advent of echocardiography, many of these cases are now being found to have mild aortic stenosis.

Revise the complications and management (in general valve replacement if symptoms present and or systolic gradient greater than 50 mm Hg). This figure is only a guide and operation may be indicated with a lower gradient if the cardiac output is low.

You may be asked the likely aetiology; remember that in a young or middle aged adult the likely cause is a congenital bicuspid valve which has become calcified; rheumatic heart disease is the next most common cause, while in elderly patients calcification in a tricuspid aortic valve may occur.

Notes

Mixed aortic regurgitation and stenosis

This is a very common case. Remember that a systolic murmur commonly occurs in aortic regurgitation even when stenosis is slight or absent.

Palpate for a bisferiens pulse (a detectable notch halfway up the upstroke).

The most reliable guide to the dominant lesion is the character of the pulse and the pulse pressure. Always ask if you may take the blood pressure for this reason.

In severe stenosis the pulse is small in volume, the blood pressure normal and the pulse pressure narrow (with occasional exceptions).

In severe regurgitation the pulse is large in volume and collapsing in nature, with a wide pulse pressure.

Notes

Tricuspid regurgitation

You must be able to recognise the prominent systolic 'cv' waves in the jugular venous pulse. Look also for a steep 'y' descent. Palpate the liver for a systolic impulse. Palpate for a left parasternal heave and feel also for a thrill in this area; auscultate for a third sound. The murmur is usually heard best at the lower left sternal edge but is sometimes clearly audible at the apex. Other valve lesions may be present, especially mitral regurgitation and/or stenosis, and these should be listened for carefully.

Mitral regurgitation is sometimes diffficult to distinguish. Of great importance in this respect is the increase in intensity of the murmur of tricuspid regurgitation on inspiration, and the presence of systolic venous pulsation. *Mitral* regurgitation is suggested by radiation of the murmur to the axilla and by left ventricular enlargement.

Listen also for a tricuspid diastolic murmur due to either high flow through the valve or concomitant stenosis.

Look for signs of right-sided heart failure, e.g. hepatic enlargement, ascites and peripheral oedema.

Seek for evidence of rare causes, especially multiple venepuncture sites (main-line drug addiction) and facial telangiectases (carcinoid syndrome). The latter disease may be associated with other right-sided heart lesions (especially pulmonary stenosis), and the patient will usually have a hard, irregular, enlarged liver due to metastases.

Revise the causes of the condition. Remember that it often occurs *secondary* to right ventricular failure.

Notes

Mitral valve prolapse

This is a popular short case, so listen to as many examples as possible during your practice sessions. You must get used to timing the late systolic murmur and/or mid-systolic click. Remember that with posterior leaflet prolapse the murmur may radiate to the left sternal edge.

In some cases the systolic murmur may be mid- or even pan-systolic; the clicks may be multiple and there may be a systolic 'squeak' or 'honk' at the apex.

Remember that most patients are otherwise normal but check for features of Marfan's syndrome in the fingers and palate. You may be asked to discuss the nature of the condition. *see Quarterly Journal of Medicine 1985 No.219 pp317-320 Oakley, C.*

It is worth noting that the effects of manoeuvres may sometimes help in distinguishing between the causes of systolic murmurs: the murmur of mitral valve prolapse is *increased* by the Valsalva manoeuvre, but *decreased* by squatting; the reverse effects occur with the manoeuvres in both mitral incompetence and aortic stenosis. See table on p.48. You are not recommended to perform these during the examination - although you may suggest them during discussion of the case if appropriate.

Notes

Hypertrophic obstructive cardiomyopathy

This is a rare short case. There is a steeply rising jerky pulse.

There may be a thrusting apex (left ventricular hypertrophy) and left parasternal heave (right ventricular hypertrophy). The murmur is a mid or late systolic ejection murmur, best heard in the left third or fourth intercostal space but occasionally maximal at the apex. An 'a' wave in the jugular venous pulse may be present, as may a fourth heart sound. The pansystolic murmur of associated mitral incompetence may occur.

Differentiation from aortic stenosis may be difficult. In HOCM there is no aortic ejection click and the second heart sound is usually normal. The murmur of HOCM radiates poorly to the carotids.

Certain 'bedside manoeuvres' may assist in the diagnosis. (*see Chester p. 258* and table below). Again you may suggest these to the examiners during discussion of the case but should not perform them routinely.

EFFECTS OF BEDSIDE MANOEUVRES ON SYSTOLIC MURMURS:

	HOCM	AS	Mitral Valve Prolapse	Mitral Regurgitation
VALSALVA	↑	↓	↑	↓
SQUATTING	↓	↑	↓	↑

Notes

Pulmonary stenosis

This condition is not infrequently shown in the membership; you must examine patients with it to become familiar with the signs.

Vital clues include the ejection click and mid-systolic murmur *loudest on inspiration*. Palpate for a thrill in the second left intercostal space, this is commonly present. In severe cases there is a left parasternal heave, the click disappears and the second sound becomes widely split with a soft second (pulmonary) element.

Remember also that the condition, although usually congenital, may be associated with carcinoid syndrome (see tricuspid regurgitation).

Another very rare association is with Kallmann's Syndrome (gonadotrophin deficiency secondary to LHRH deficiency with anosmia); other congenital defects may coexist.

Notes

Atrial septal defect

This will usually be of the ostium secundum variety.

The pulse volume may be small and there may be a left parasternal heave due to right ventricular hypertrophy.

You must get used to hearing the wide split second sound, not varying with respiration: practice is the only way to do this. Having heard the split second sound always listen carefully at the second left intercostal space for the common ejection systolic murmur due to high flow through the pulmonary valve. There may also be a tricuspid mid-diastolic flow murmur at the lower left sternal edge which will be louder on inspiration.

In the rare ostium primum variety, murmurs of associated lesions (mitral and/or tricuspid regurgitation) may be present.

Look for evidence of pulmonary hypertension (see Eisenmenger's Syndrome) and revise the complications of the condition.

Notes

Ventricular septal defect

A fairly common short case. The pulse volume may be small if there is a large left to right shunt. There may be a thrill at the lower left sternal edge and a loud 'tearing' pansystolic murmur maximal at this site. Listen also for a mid-diastolic murmur at the apex due to high flow through the mitral valve.

Look for evidence of complications:

* pulmonary hypertension, leading eventually to Eisenmenger's Syndrome (NB pansystolic murmur may soften in this case, see p.52)
* biventricular failure
* endocarditis (look for splinter haemorrhages)

Remember that a *small* defect may produce a *loud* murmur (Maladie de Roger).

Notes

Eisenmenger's syndrome

In this case you will usually be presented with a patient who is centrally cyanosed and clubbed and you will be asked to examine the cardiovascular system. The pulse volume will usually be small. Look for signs of pulmonary hypertension and right ventricular hypertrophy on palpation:

* left parasternal heave
* palpable pulmonary valve closure (pulmonary diastolic shock)

Auscultate for a loud second sound, right ventricular fourth sound, pulmonary efection click, and early diastolic murmur of pulmonary regurgitation +/– pansystolic murmur of tricuspid regurgitation.

Attempt to identify the cause of the syndrome (often very difficult):

* atrial septal defect there will be a fixed split second sound

* in ventricular septal defect the characteristic pansystolic murmur may become soft or disappear, while the second sound may become single (equal pressure in both ventricles)

* in persistent ductus arteriosus the second sound remains normally split: differential cyanosis is diagnostic. (The venous blood is shunted into the decending aorta so that only the lower limbs become cyanosed i.e. differential cyanosis).

Notes

Coarctation of the aorta

An uncommon short case. Remember that the constriction is usually just distal to the origin of the left subclavian artery (near the insertion of the ligamentum arteriosum).

Early clues to the lesion on inspection may be greater development of the upper extremities and thorax than the lower extremities and (sometimes) visible scapular collaterals. Usually, however, the first evidence comes from testing for radiofemoral delay, which should therefore be a routine part of your cardiovascular examination. On occasion the left subclavian artery is involved and there may be asymmetrical radial pulses (see p.36).

Palpate for a thrusting apex (left ventricular hypertrophy) and listen for the systolic murmur of the coarctation, both anteriorly and posteriorly, over the left upper thorax. Listen also for aortic systolic and (occasionally) diastolic murmurs from an associated bicuspid aortic valve, and listen for murmurs of collaterals over the scapulae. Revise the complications and associations of the condition.

Notes

Pericarditis

Occasionally a patient with a pericardial friction rub is shown as a short case, the candidate being asked to "Examine the precordium".

Revise the causes of this.

Cardiac tamponade and constrictive pericarditis are most unlikely to occur as short cases though you should revise the signs.

Notes

Prosthetic heart valves

Patients with metallic prosthetic aortic or mitral valves are sometimes shown as short cases and you must be able to distinguish between them.

Their characteristic sounds are summarised below. Note that 'pig' valves do not produce these sounds.

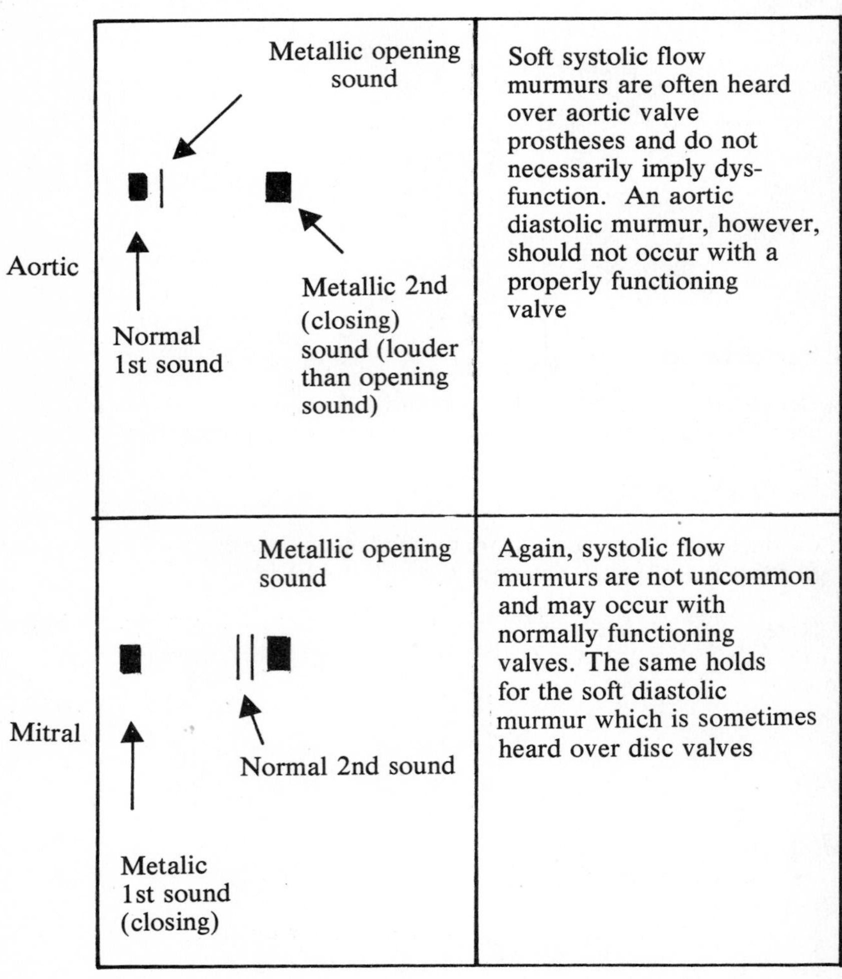

The closing sound is the dominant one with both valves and, by timing this in relation to the carotid pulse, it should be possible to identify rapidly which valve is prosthetic (beware, they may both be!).

Disc valves tend to make a 'clicking' noise on opening or closing while ball and cage valves have a characteristic 'plopping' sound.

Remember that complications of valve replacement include valve leakage or mechanical dysfunction, endocarditis, thromboembolism, bleeding due to anticoagulants and haemolytic anaemia.

Notes

Infective endocarditis

Not common as a short case but *always* check for splinter haemorrhages* and clubbing in every cardiovascular examination.

The latter sign implies chronic disease and is less likely to be found in modern practice.

If you suspect the diagnosis look further at the hands for:

Osler's nodes*
Janeway lesions*

Look for petechial rashes* on the skin and conjunctivae.
Look at the conjunctivae for evidence of anaemia.

Palpate for splenomegaly (40%).

Examine the fundi for Roth's spots*.

Tell the examiner that you would like to test the urine for microscopic haematuria and/or proteinuria. Say also that you would normally proceed to examine the chest and limbs for evidence of pulmonary or cerebral embolism.

Revise the clinical features of the condition (in terms of signs due to):

a) Infection
b) Embolism
c) Immune complex disease
d) Cardiac Disease *(see Medicine International, vol.2 Sept 1985 No.21 pp.872-888, C. Oakley).*

Remember that right sided lesions (especially tricuspid and pulmonary regurgitation) occur in main-line drug addicts (look for multiple venepuncture sites) who usually have no predisposing cardiac lesions.

Remember also that the pattern of the disease is changing with a tendency for more acute than subacute forms to occur.

*Immune complex phenomena. Glomerulonephritis and neuropsychiatric manifestations may be due to either emboli or immune complex mediated vasculitis.

Notes

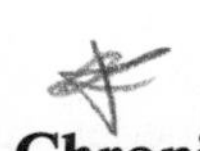

RESPIRATORY SHORT CASES

Chronic bronchitis/emphysema

This is a common short case and you must have a method of examination fully prepared in order to be able to shine.

1. Always start by examining the sputum pot.

2. Look at the nails for nicotine staining or clubbing (the latter suggests pathology other than emphysema or chronic bronchitis).

3. Feel the hands and pulse for signs of carbon dioxide retention (e.g. warm hands, rapid bounding pulse).

4. Look at the face and conjunctivae for plethora, and at the underside of the tongue and vermilion border of the lip for central cyanosis.

5. Observe the patient from the end of the bed: count the respiratory rate and look for purse-lip breathing.

6. Examine carefully for evidence of hyperinflation of the chest:

   a) Symmetrical diminution of chest expansion.
   b) Increased A-P diameter of the chest (but note this may also occur in disorders of the thoracic spine).
   c) Use of accessory muscles of respiration; especially the sternocleidomastoids (also scaleni, trapezii).
   d) Indrawing of intercostal spaces, supraclavicular fossae and costal margins on inspiration.
   e) Shortening of the distance between the cricoid cartilage and the suprasternal notch to less than 3 finger-breadths. Trachea may descend on inspiration.
   f) Loss of cardiac and hepatic dullness. The apex beat may be impalpable (other causes: obesity, pencardial effusion, dextrocardia).
   g) Hyperresonance of the chest on percussion.

The breath sounds may be quiet: remember that early inspiratory crackles especially at the bases, frequently occur in chronic bronchitis, as do expiratory wheezes.

Look for elevation of the jugular venous pulse and ankle oedema which may suggest right-sided heart failure (cor pulmonale).

Try to decide whether your patient fits into the category of 'pink puffer' or 'blue bloater' (see chart below) or whether he has features of both. If you suspect CO_2 retention, ask if you may examine the fundi for papilloedema, and test for flapping tremor of the outstretched hands.

	Pink Puffer	Blue Bloater
Build	Thin	Obese
Cyanosis	–	+
Breathlessness	++	+
Hyperinflation of chest	+++	+
Cor pulmonale	–	+ (often)

Notes

Bronchiectasis

This condition is quite commonly shown as a short case. There may be evidence of copious sputum production, sometimes blood-stained, in the sputum pot on the bedside locker: always inspect this first.

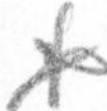
The patient is often clubbed.

The characteristic finding is of coarse, leathery crackles, often over the bases; during acute exacerbations there may be a pleural rub.

If you are reasonably confident of the diagnosis you may go on to look for dextrocardia (present, with sinusitis, in Kartagener's syndrome) and ask whether you may examine for features of secondary amyloidosis (e.g. hepatosplenomegaly).

Revise the causes of the condition *(see Flenley, p.135),* but remember to mention common causes like childhood measles or whooping cough and cystic fibrosis before rarer ones such as hypogammaglobulinaemia.

Notes

Fibrosing alveolitis

This is a popular short case, with which you must be familiar.

The patient is usually clubbed. In advanced cases central cyanosis is present at rest. Chest expansion is limited and the percussion note may be dull over the lower thorax due to elevation of the diaphragm as the lung volume shrinks.

The hallmark of the disease is the presence of showers of bilateral fine basal crackles in late inspiration; characteristically they become quieter or disappear when the patient leans forward. Unlike the crackles of pulmonary oedema (which may also be late inspiratory) they do not clear on coughing; test for this.

Look for evidence of pulmonary hypertension (loud P_2, 'a' waves in jugular venous pulse, left parasternal heave) and cor pulmonale (raised JVP, tender hepatomegaly, peripheral oedema). Note that these occur only late in the disease course.

Occasionally there will be evidence of diseases associated with fibrosing alveolitis (e.g. rheumatoid arthritis, systemic lupus erythematosus, systemic sclerosis, dermatomyositis (*see Medicine International Vol.1 1982.No.22 p.1020 A. Johnson.*) Remember the causes of clubbing with basal crackles: fibrosing alveolitis, bronchiectasis, asbestosis. Carcinoma should of course always be considered in a clubbed patient with respiratory disease.

Notes

Pleural effusion

A common short case. Occasionally needlemarks from diagnostic or therapeutic aspiration are present.

Remember to percuss and auscultate into the axillae. Listen for bronchial breathing and test for aegophony at the upper level of an effusion.

It will not usually be possible to suggest the underlying cause of the effusion although you should look for clues e.g. signs of cardiac failure; clubbing and cachexia (suggesting bronchial carcinoma); rheumatoid hands; butterfly rash of systemic lupus erythematosus.

Revise the causes in terms of transudates and exudates.

Notes

Pneumonia

With increasing emphasis on acute cases in the examination you should be prepared to examine patients with (usually resolving) pneumonia.Revise the signs.

Notes

Pulmonary fibrosis

Patients with apical fibrosis commonly appear as short cases and you must be able to demonstrate the signs confidently.

The chest may be flattened over an area of fibrosis; this and tracheal deviation towards the affected side are vital clues. Expansion will be reduced on the affected side and the percussion note dull. Remember that low-pitched bronchial breathing may be heard over an area of fibrosis.

Always look carefully for scars: patient may have had one of the operations for tuberculosis performed more commonly in the past: plombage; thoracoplasty; phrenic nerve crush; artificial pneumothorax.
Patients who have had a lobectomy may also be shown.

Note: although most cases of apical fibrosis are tuberculous in origin, radiotherapy is an important cause to remember (look for markings).

Rarely, ankylosing spondylitis may cause apical fibrosis (see p.128).

Notes

Superior vena caval obstruction

A rare 'spot diagnosis' case. You may be asked to observe the patient from the end of the bed. The patient is often tachypnoeic.

You must be able to recognise the characteristic suffused and oedematous appearance of the face, neck and arms; there are dilated and tortuous veins on the anterior chest wall and upper limbs. There is non-pulsatile elevation of the jugular venous pressure. If the obstruction is due to bronchial carcinoma (as is often the case), the markings for radiotherapy may be visible. Much rarer causes include enlargement of the thyroid or thymus glands.

Notes

ABDOMINAL SHORT CASES

You must be absolutely precise in your method of examination and description of the liver, spleen, kidneys and any abdominal mass.

Watch the patient's face to make sure you do not hurt him during the examination.

Hepatomegaly

Always percuss out the upper and lower borders of the liver (the upper border is normally in the fifth intercostal space but may be displaced downwards if the patient has emphysema).

Describe any enlargement in centimetres (easily measured with a pocket ruler) or finger breadths below the costal margin. Comment on the *edge, surface, consistency, tenderness, and pulsation*.

Auscultate for a bruit over the liver (heard in hepatoma and occasionally alcoholic hepatitis). A friction rub may occur with malignant deposits. If the liver is pulsatile look for other signs of tricuspid regurgitation (see p.46)

Having found hepatomegaly you must proceed with the remainder of the abdominal examination, looking especially for *splenomegaly, ascites, and lymphadenopathy* - whose presence or absence alters the differential diagnosis (see hepatosplenomegaly).

Remember the possibility of a Riedl's lobe (more common in women) which may extend laterally down as far as the right lumbar region.

You should now spend a few seconds glancing for peripheral clues in the hands (see p.70), eyes (? jaundice, ? xanthelasmata, ? Kayser-Fleischer rings), jugular venous pulse (? elevated - suggests right ventricular failure) and skin (? pigmented as in haemachromatosis or primary biliary cirrhosis; ? scratch marks, ? spider naevi (prominent in primary biliary cirrhosis). Do *not* spend long doing this, however, as you may waste time and irritate the examiners.

List the causes of hepatomegaly. Remember that *common* causes include:

* Congestive cardiac failure.
* Cirrhosis (but note that liver may become impalpable in advanced cases).
* Carcinomatosis.
* Infections (e.g. infective hepatitis, infectious mononucleosis).

Revise the physical features of the liver in each of these cases.

Popular examination cases to remember are haemochromatosis and primary biliary cirrhosis (see p.72)

Notes

Splenomegaly

A common short case used to test your skills of abdominal examination.

Always start palpation in the right iliac fossa to avoid missing massive splenomegaly. A spleen 'tip' may be better felt with the patient rolled onto his right side with the left arm extended and the left hip and knee flexed.

You will almost invariably be asked to justify your diagnosis in terms of the classical signs:

* Dull to percussion (continuous with area of splenic dullness over 9th, 10th and 11th ribs in midaxillary line)
* Enlarges obliquely towards right lower quadrant
* Distinct edge with medial notch may be palpable
* Downward movement on inspiration
* Cannot palpate above the swelling.

You must have an organised list of causes of massive, moderate and slight splenomegaly at your fingertips. A suggested scheme is outlined below but you should expand this or devise your own for ease of memorising. Remember to give the causes common *in this country* first e.g. myelofibrosis, rather than kala-azar, for massive splenomegaly.

Massive	(> 8 cm)	: myelofibrosis, chronic myeloid leukaemia, malaria, kala-azar, Gaucher's disease.
Moderate	(4-8 cm)	: the above plus haemolytic anaemias, lymphoproliferative disease, portal hypertension.
Slight	(4 cm)	: all the above plus infections (NB infectious mononucleosis, infective endocarditis), blood disorders (e.g. polycythaemia rubra vera, idiopathic thrombocytopenic purpura, pernicious anaemia, systemic lupus erythematosus, sarcoidosis, amyloidosis, Felty's syndrome).

Remember that, as always, if you mention a rare disease, you may be asked to discuss it.

Notes

Hepatosplenomegaly

A very common short case. As always your technique for demonstrating enlargement of the organs must be quick and accurate. Proceed swiftly to complete your abdominal examination and look carefully for signs of ascites, chronic liver disease and especially generalised lymphadenopathy (examine inguinal, axillary, cervical and supraclavicular regions).

As leukaemias are a common cause of hepatosplenomegaly, test for sternal tenderness if you suspect this diagnosis.

You will be asked the differential diagnosis in your patient: the following is intended as a guide to some common causes: you should expand it yourself as a revision exercise.

LIVER + SPLEEN	Chronic Myeloid Leukaemia / Myelofibrosis } usually SPLEEN ++ LIVER + Lymphoproliferative disorders - usually SPLEEN+ LIVER+ (superficial nodes may not be palpable even when mediastinal or retroperitoneal nodes are enlarged) NB Cirrhosis + portal hypertension may exist without ascites but signs of chronic liver disease will be present In a young patient remember β-thalassaemia major: usually LIVER++ SPLEEN++. Look for slate-grey skin (iron deposition) and bossed skull.
LIVER + SPLEEN + NODES	Lymphoproliferative disorders: Chronic lymphocytic leukaemia / Lymphoma Rarer causes always worth including in your differential diagnosis are: Systemic lupus erythematosus (look for butterfly rash) Sarcoidosis (look for skin lesions).
SPLEEN + LYMPH NODES	As for liver, spleen + nodes but remember Infections: Acute e.g. Infectious mononucleosis / Chronic e.g. Tuberculosis, brucellosis Felty's Syndrome (popular in examinations, look for rheumatoid hands)

<table>
<tr>
<td>ISOLATED

SPLENO-
MEGALY</td>
<td>Infections e.g. septicaemia
infective endocarditis (look for splinter haemorrhages)

typhoid

Haematological causes:

Haemolytic anaemia (e.g. Hereditary spherocytosis; anaemia + jaundice present)

Myelofibrosis } spleen may
CML } be massive

Lymphoma

Idiopathic thrombocytopenic purpura (anaemia + purpura present)

Polycythaemia rubra vera (plethoric face)

Cirrhosis + portal hypertension: liver may be impalpable but signs of chronic liver disease usually present.</td>
</tr>
</table>

Notes

Renal enlargement

Patients with bilateral renal enlargement are commonly shown in the short cases. The usual cause is polycystic kidney disease: the kidneys may sometimes be grossly enlarged and can even meet in the middle.
Rarer causes include bilateral hydronephrosis and amyloidosis. If you suspect polycystic kidneys you should ask to take the blood pressure (raised in over 50% of cases). Revise the other complications of this condition. *(See Gabriel).* Having diagnosed a mass as a kidney you must be able to support this with your physical findings:

* Bimanually palpable
* Ballotable
* Resonant to percussion
* Examining hand can get between swelling and costal margin
* Slight movement downwards on inspiration.

Remember that the lower pole of the normal right kidney is often palpable in slim people.

Some patients with polycystic disease of the kidneys also have a polycystic liver which may be palpable. Another association is with berry aneurysms (remember that a posterior communicating artery aneurysm may cause a third nerve palsy; look for this).

Unilateral renal enlargement is less commonly shown (causes include renal cyst, carcinoma, hydronephrosis or hypertrophy of a single functioning kidney).

Notes

Ascites

Remember the five causes of abdominal distension (fat, fluid, flatus, faeces, fetus; according to rumour the last of these has appeared in the clinical on at least one occasion!). Practise your method of testing for shifting dullness and a fluid thrill. Always percuss with the finger on the abdomen parallel to the border of the fluid - you will not be able to locate the limit of the ascites otherwise. In the examination ascites is likely to be found in the context of cirrhosis and portal hypertension or abdominal malignancy. Revise the list of causes of ascites, dividing them into transudates and exudates and be able to discuss the investigation and management of a case. *(See Sherlock, Chapter 10.)*

Notes

Chronic liver disease

This is a very popular case, with numerous signs to be found. The candidate is usually asked to "Examine the abdominal system".

Peripheral signs should be *briefly* looked for as they often give an early clue as to the diagnosis. Look carefully at:

The hands: clubbing, leuconychia, palmar erythema (NB Other causes of palmar erythema include rheumatoid arthritis, pregnancy, chronic leukaemia and thyrotoxicosis), Dupuytren's contracture, spider naevi (more than five is pathological), 'liver flap'.

The face: spider naevi, telangiectasia (paper money skin). jaundice, pigmentation (especially in PBC and haemochromatosis) central cyanosis (one third of patients with decompensated cirrhosis have reduced arterial oxygen saturation due to intrapulmonary shunting through AV fistulae *(New Eng. J. Med. 263, 73, 1960)*, hepatic foetor, bilateral parotid enlargement.

The limbs: ankle oedema, muscle wasting, bruising.

The trunk: loss of axillary, chest and pubic hair, gynaecomastia, excoriations.

Examine the abdomen: Examine especially for hepatomegaly and signs of portal hypertension: splenomegaly ascites and prominent periumbilical veins (flow in these collaterals is uniformly away from the umbilicus, unlike the situation in inferior venal caval obstruction where the flow in collateral vessels is uniformly upwards).

If the liver is impalpable percuss for contraction of the organ (only present in cirrhosis or fulminant hepatic failure). Auscultate over the umbilicus for a venous hum and over the liver for a systolic bruit (which may suggest development of hepatoma).

Remember that signs of 'decompensation' include flapping tremor* of the hands (asterixis) - demonstrate with the wrists dorsiflexed, hepatic foetor, development of encephalopathy (constructional apraxia, e.g. inability to copy the drawing of a 'star', is a useful sign) and jaundice. You should comment on their presence or absence.

* NB A flapping tremor can also be seen in uraemia, respiratory failure or severe heart failure.

Notes

Special cases of chronic liver disease

a) Primary biliary cirrhosis

Consider this in a pigmented patient with prominent excoriations (due to marked pruritus). Look carefully for xanthelasmata and xanthomata over joints, skinfolds and sites of trauma (including venepuncture). Finger clubbing is common and should be looked for. The spleen is often palpable (50% of cases).

Remember that steatorrhea in the condition may lead to easy bruising, osteoporosis and osteomalacia (test for tenderness over the spine).

Important associations of the condition include: rheumatoid arthritis, dermatomyositis, autoimmune thyroiditis, the CREST syndrome (calcinosis, Raynaud's phenomenon, oesophageal dysfunction, sclerodactyly and telangiectasia), Sjogren's syndrome and renal tubular acidosis.

Notes

b) Haemochromatosis

The patient is typically a middle-aged male with slate-grey skin pigmentation, maximal in exposed parts, groins, axillae, genitalia and old scars (due to *melanin*) and a characteristically large and firm liver. The spleen is usually palpable but portal hypertension, ascites and hepatocellular failure are rare. Loss of secondary sexual hair is often prominent.

If you suspect the diagnosis, look for signs of arthropathy (due to pyrophosphate and affecting two thirds of patients) in the metacarpophalangeal and larger joints.

Tell the examiner that you would like to examine:

a) the cardiovascular system (for signs of heart failure)
b) the urine for glucose (clinical diabetes in 66% of patients)
c) the genitalia (for testicular atrophy).

Notes

c) Chronic active hepatitis

In this case the patient is usually a young female. Notable features include a cushingoid appearance, acne, hirsutism, cutaneous striae and vascular spiders. The spleen is usually enlarged, even in the absence of portal hypertension.

Revise the associations *(see Medicine International Vol. 1 No. 16, p. 726 S. Sherlock.)*

Notes

Abdominal masses

List and revise the causes of masses in each segment of the abdomen.

Any mass which you find must be fully described in terms of site, size, shape, surface, mobility, pulsatility, percussion note and presence or absence of a bruit.

Many masses are visible on careful observation of the abdomen - never neglect this vital step. Common sources of difficulty include:

1. **Epigastric masses:** important causes include gastric carcinoma (check for left supraclavicular nodes (Troisier's sign/Virchow's nodes) and pancreatic pseudocyst. Two 'catches' are:

   a) left lobe of liver. Furthermore a post-necrotic nodule in a cirrhotic liver may simulate a gastric mass.
   b) large rectus muscles: these will seem to enlarge if the patient is asked to sit forwards.

   Occasionally large retroperitoneal nodes (in lymphoma) may be palpable in the epigastrium or umbilical region.

2. **Suprapubic masses:** these are often missed: always remember to palpate in this area. A most important sign of pelvic masses is that their lower limit is not palpable. As well as the urinary bladder remember the possibility of an enlarged uterus (e.g. fibroids) or ovarian cyst (frequently palpable in the midline) in female patients.

3. **Left and right iliac fossae:** masses in the abdomen are not the sole property of the surgeons: you should be able to give a differential diagnosis. The following is an abbreviated list: you will find it useful to expand it yourself to include the rarer causes.

RIGHT ILIAC FOSSA	LEFT ILIAC FOSSA
Carcinoma of caecum Crohn's disease Appendix mass	Carcinoma of colon* Diverticular abscess
Less common Iliocaecal T.B. Ovarian cyst Pelvic (or transplanted) kidney Iliac lymphadenopathy	Less common Crohn's disease Ovarian cyst Pelvic (or transplanted) kidney Iliac lymphadenopathy *NB Normal descending and sigmoid colon is often palpable especially if loaded with faeces

Notes

Right upper quadrant masses

Masses in this area include hepatic (including Riedl's lobe), renal, and colonic swellings; and occasionally an enlarged gallbladder (revise Courvoisier's law and state this if the patient is jaundiced). It is sometimes difficult to distinguish between these masses and in this case you should state your findings followed by a differential diagnosis. You may be asked how you would investigate the patient: mention simple tests first (e.g. urine testing for blood or protein, faecal occult blood, plain abdominal X-rays followed by ultrasound scan: further tests may include barium enema, liver scan, IVP as appropriate).

Aortic aneurysm

Remember that the abdominal aorta bifurcates at the level of the umbilicus and may be easily palpable in thin patients.

Always test for *expansile* pulsation which is present with aortic aneurysm but not if the pulsation is being transmitted.
Auscultate over the swelling, a loud bruit (in the absence of a similar bruit in the heart) supports the diagnosis of aneurysm.

Notes

NEUROLOGICAL SHORT CASES

The examination of neurological short cases requires a great deal of polish and confidence which can only be achieved through practice. It is certainly a great advantage to have done a neurology job and if you have not done so, it might be worth considering attending one of the special courses on neurology for the Membership. In any case, you must devote plenty of time to neurological cases during your practice sessions.

Visual field defects

Revise the causes of the following field defects which occasionally appear as short cases:

	Notes
Homonymous hemianopia	
Bitemporal hemianopia	
Central scotoma	
Concentric constriction.	

Remember that a homonymous hemianopia, the commonest case, implies a lesion posterior to the optic chiasm (in the optic tract, radiation or occipital cortex). Note the following:

* A lesion in the anterior occipital cortex (e.g. due to posterior cerebral artery occlusion) causes a macular sparing hemianopia; *(see Patten p.19)*
* Lesions in the optic tract may lead to an incongruous hemianopia.
* Lesions of the optic radiation may produce an upper quadrantic hemianopia with a temporal lobe lesion, or a lower quadrantic hemianopia with a parietal lobe lesion.

PUPILLARY ABNORMALITIES

Horner's syndrome

This is a very common short case, "Look at this man's eyes".

* The ptosis and meiosis should be readily apparent. Check for the other features: enophthalmos and loss of forehead sweating on the same side. In congenital cases the iris remains blue/grey; look for this.

* Test the reactions to light and accommodation, these should be present and normal.

* Proceed to inspect the neck for scars from cervical sympathectomy (a common short case) or thyroidectomy.

* Palpate for cervical ribs and cervical lymphadenopathy.

* Examine for weakness of the small muscles of the hand (T1) and for loss of sensation over the T1 dermatome (T1 involvement, commonly due to Pancoast's syndrome).

* Test for loss of pain and temperature in the arm and face, loss of arm reflexes, bulbar palsy and nystagmus (syringomyelia/syringobulbia).

* Tell the examiner that you would like to examine the chest clinically and radiologically for evidence of Pancoast's tumour.

* Revise the list of causes of the syndrome according to their anatomical level:

  i.e. Hemisphere
  Brain stem
  Cervical cord
  T1 root
  Sympathetic chain.

(see Patten p. 7).

Notes

Holmes-Adie pupil

The patient is often a healthy young female; the unilateral dilated pupil is striking. The eye is in the normal position with no ptosis.

* Look for ptosis and test ocular movements for evidence of third nerve palsy (the main alternative diagnosis).
* Test the response to light (very slow) and accommodation (also slow but more definite).
* Ask the examiner's permission to test the knee jerks (often absent).

Remember that the Holmes-Adie pupil constricts promptly to 2.5% methacholine. However a word of warning: another cause of unilateral dilated pupil (usually fixed to light and accommodation) is mydriatic eye drops!

Notes

Fundi

Revise the following popular examination cases by sketching the characteristic appearances in the spaces below:

Diabetic retinopathy a) background	b) proliferative	c) malignant hypertension
d) optic atrophy	e) choroiditis	f) retinitis pigmentosa
g) retinal artery thrombosis	h) retinal vein thrombosis	i) angioid streaks
j) senile macular degeneration	k) papilloedema	l) glaucoma

Notes on fundi

a) **Diabetes**: you will be expected to comment on whether the retinopathy is background or proliferative. Remember that in the latter condition as well as new vessel formation, there may be the complications of vitreous haemorrhage, fibrous tissue formation, retinal detachment and rubeosis iridis (which may in turn lead to glaucoma). Laser burns will often be present.

b) **Hypertensive retinopathy**: the case will usually be of malignant hypertension. Revise the Keith, Wagener and Barber classification (less used now than before, but you may be expected to know it):

Grade 1. Arteriolar narrowing/silver-wiring

Grade 2. AV nipping

Grade 3. Haemorrhages + exudates (soft / hard)

Grade 4. As for 3, but with papilloedema.

c) **Optic atrophy**: divide the causes into

primary (direct damage to nerve, e.g. post neuritic, optic nerve compression, ischaemic, traumatic, toxic, infective (e.g. syphilis), malnutritional or hereditary (e.g. Leber's): disc is very pale with distinct lamina cribrosa;

secondary (after papilloedema): the disc is grey-white with indistinct edges and lamina cribrosa;

consecutive to retinal disease, e.g. retinitis pigmentosa, choroiditis.

d) **Choroiditis**:irregular areas of white sclera with dark patches of pigment-epithelium. Note: laser burns may give similar appearance. Toxoplasmosis is a common and important cause; revise the others.

e) **Retinitis pigmentosa**: be sure that you can recognise this classic case. As well as occurring as an isolated abnormality, it may be associated with a variety of hereditary syndromes, e.g.

Laurence Moon-Biedl (polydactyly, obesity, mental retardation), Refsum's disease (see p.87). There may be concentric field constriction;

NB night vision is lost early. *(see Kritzinger and Wright p.14)*

f) **Retinal artery thrombosis** remember that a 'cherry red spot' may be seen at the macula (choroid visible through this retina) from one to two days after the occlusion: in late cases there is optic atrophy. Revise the associations.

g) **Retinal vein occlusion** branch or central vein occlusions may be shown. In the latter there may be papilloedema. *(see Kritzinger and Wright p.49)*

h) **Angioid streaks** occur classically in pseudoxanthoma elasticaum. Look for chicken-skin lesions on the neck: yellowish papules forming plaques with loss of elasticity. Axillae, elbows and groins are other sites for these. They may also occur in Paget's disease and sickle-cell anaemia. The defect is in Bruch's membrane. *(see Kritzinger and Wright p.16.)*

i) **Senile macular degeneration**: macula may be mottled with pigment or swollen with exudate or contain haemorrhagic residues.

j) **Papilloedema**: revise the progressive changes occurring in its development *(see Patten p.27).* Note that the disc may appear pink in optic neuritis, but in this case there is usually marked loss of visual acuity and pain on moving the eye.

k) **Glaucoma**: the deeply cupped disc may be shown. Remember that cupping and pallor may occur in myopia, while hypermetropia may cause small, pink discs (pseudopapilloedema).

Notes

Ocular palsies

These are commonly shown ("Examine these eyes" or "This man has double vision, would you examine his eyes?").

On inspection third and sixth nerve palsies may be obvious. You must quickly demonstrate which muscles are weak and the direction in which reported diplopia is maximal. In less obvious cases you should be able to analyse the diplopia by using the cover test (when looking in the direction of action of the weak muscle, the outer image disappears on covering the affected eye).

In the case of a third nerve palsy you must state whether the lesion is complete or partial. In a *complete* lesion there is complete ptosis, the eye is deviated downwards and outwards with loss of upward, downward and medial movements, and a dilated, unreactive pupil. It is obviously necessary to elevate the eyelid to observe the latter findings because of the ptosis. Note that in vascular lesions of the third nerve (e.g. in diabetes, arteriosclerosis or arteritis) the pupil may be spared.

You should demonstrate whether the fourth nerve is intact by lifting the eyelid and asking the patient to look down: if the nerve is intact there will be intorsion of the eye (*see Patten p.23*). Test lateral gaze to confirm that the sixth nerve is intact.

You may be asked the likely cause: remember that the commonest causes of a *pure* third nerve palsy are posterior communicating artery aneurysm, diabetes, atherosclerosis, and raised intracranial pressure.
The latter three are also common causes of a sixth nerve palsy.

Revise a full list of causes of ocular palsies, dividing them into lesions in the brain stem, base of skull, cavernous sinus and orbit.

Remember that the third, fourth and sixth nerves may be affected singly or in combination as part of a *cranial neuropathy* due to:

Diabetes
Polyarteritis nodosa
Multiple sclerosis
Sarcoidosis
Basal meningitis: tuberculous, syphilitic, carcinomatous

There are two traps to be wary of:

1. Congenital squint: the eyes move together, the angle between their longitudinal axis remaining constant.

2. Dysthyroid eye disease and myasthenia gravis: both may produce *complex* eye signs due to involvement of the eye muscles. Always look for exophthalmos, a goitre or thyroid scar, or (in myasthenia) bilateral ptosis.

There is an excellent illustrated account of ocular palsies in *A Colour Atlas of Clinical Neurology. Parsons M. 1983. Wolfe Medical Publications Ltd.*

Notes

Nystagmus

You will usually be asked to "Examine these eyes" and you must always look carefully for nystagmus, both on horizontal and on vertical gaze (candidates often miss the latter through failing to observe specifically for it). Remember to keep within the range of binocular vision and wait for at least 5 seconds in each position. Describe the nystagmus in terms of its type, direction of fast phase and maximal amplitude. Note that in vestibular nystagmus the fast phase is away from the side of the lesion, while in cerebellar nystagmus the opposite is true. Brainstem nystagmus is typically multidirectional, and may be *vertical* or *rotary*.

Remember that pendular nystagmus (a rare short case: look for pink eyes of albinism) is associated with poor visual acuity.

Some neurologists also grade nystagmus into:

Grade 1: present on looking in one direction only.

Grade 2: present with the eyes in the neutral position.

Grade 3: present on looking to either side.

Be able to give the common causes of nystagmus.

Ataxic nystagmus is a popular case so be sure that you can demonstrate the signs (nystagmus greater in abducting eye often with associated weakness of adduction due to internuclear ophthalmoplegia): NB the lesion is in the median longitudinal bundle and strongly suggests multiple sclerosis.

When you have completed your examination of the eyes (remember to check for optic atrophy, which is often present if the patient has multiple sclerosis), you may ask permission to look for signs elsewhere to elucidate the cause. In particular, it may be helpful to test for cerebellar signs (e.g. finger-nose test), test the hearing (e.g. Menière's disease) and inspect the tympanic membrane for evidence of otitis media.

Notes

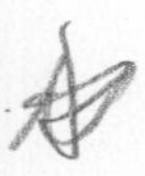

Facial nerve palsy

You must be able to distinguish between upper and lower motor neurone lesions of the seventh nerve, as well as having lists of their causes ready.

You must be able to demonstrate the global unilateral facial weakness present after a lower motor neurone lesion (a common case, usually due to Bell's palsy). Have a series of commands ready, for example: "raise your eyebrows like this", "wrinkle your forehead like this", "smile", "show me your teeth", "whistle".

* Palpate for parotid enlargement (the seventh nerve may be involved in malignant tumour).

* Inspect the external auditory meatus and fauces for vesicles (Ramsay-Hunt syndrome) and the tympanic membrane for evidence of otitis media (a rare cause today).

* Tell the examiner that you would like to ask the patient whether he has become intolerant to high-pitched or loud sounds (hyperacusis due to paralysis of stapaedius muscle) and that you would normally test taste sensation on the anterior two thirds of the tongue (involvement of chorda tympani).

In a patient with *bilateral* lower motor neurone facial weakness consider Guillain-Barré syndrome and sarcoidosis (bilateral Bell's palsy is very rare).

Notes

Peripheral neuropathy

This is a common short case: you should be able to demonstrate the symmetrical peripheral diminution of sensation to all modalities +/- motor weakness. Diminution or absence of reflexes is a most important finding; always test again with reinforcement.

* Look for trophic changes and Charcot's joints. Common causes of the latter are diabetes mellitus, syringomyelia (especially shoulder joint)

* Palpate for tenderness of affected muscles which is common in diabetic or alcoholic polyneuropathy. Palpate for *thickened peripheral nerves* present in:

Amyloidosis

Refsum's disease (cerebellar damage, peripheral neuropathy, deafness and retinitis pigmentosa)

Leprosy

Dejerine-Sottas disease (hypertrophic peripheral neuropathy)

Charcot-Marie Tooth disease (peroneal muscular atrophy) some thickening detectable in 25% of cases. *(Ref: Patten.)*

* Glance briefly for clues as to the cause:

Insulin injection sites (diabetes mellitus)

Signs of chronic liver disease (espicially alcoholic)

Anaemia + slight jaundice (B_{12} deficiency, but note that neuropathy may occur without haematological disturbance)

Cachexia (malignancy)

Pigmentation, anaemia + brown line on nails +/—

evidence of haemodialysis (uraemia)

Pes cavus (peroneal muscular atrophy or Friedreich's ataxia)

Rheumatoid hands, or butterfly rash of systemic lupus erythematosus.

Remember that a predominantly *motor neuropathy* occurs in:

Guillain-Barré syndrome
Peroneal muscular atrophy
Lead poisoning
Porphyria.

A predominantly sensory neuropathy often occurs in:

Diabetes mellitus
Malignancy (especially Ca bronchus)
Vitamin B_{12} and B_1 deficiency
Chronic renal failure
Leprosy.

Remember that the combination of peripheral neuropathy with cranial nerve involvement may occur in diabetes mellitus, sarcoidosis, Guillain-Barré syndrome (especially bilateral LMN VII palsy) and polyarteritis. *(Ref: Prout and Cooper p.188).*

Revise the causes of mononeuritis multiplex.

The following peripheral nerve lesions are occasionally shown as short cases: make notes on the signs which you would look for with lesions at different levels of the following *(see Patten p.200-203).*

Ulnar nerve lesion

Usually due to lesion at the elbow; inspect for scars or arthritis.

Occasionally due to repeated trauma to heel of hand (no sensory loss in this case).

Notes

Median nerve lesion

Carpal tunnel syndrome is a common case (NB associations include pregnancy, myxoedema, rheumatoid arthritis, acromegaly, trauma). Remember that sensory loss is very variable and that the palm is spared since the palmar branch of the medial nerve passes superficial to the flexor retinaculum.

Notes

Radial nerve lesion

Notes

a) Axilla

b) Spiral groove (spares triceps and triceps reflex)

c) Posterior interosseous nerve

Unilateral foot-drop

Here the main differential diagnosis is between:

a) Pyramidal lesion affecting lower limb (e.g. cerebrovascular accident; multiple sclerosis: pyramidal weakness, hyperreflexia and upgoing plantar should make diagnosis obvious).

b) Common peroneal nerve palsy; weakness of dorsiflexion of feet and toes and of *eversion of foot*. Ankle jerk is intact and plantar response normal; sensory loss often *restricted* to dorsum of foot (may extend to anterolateral aspect of leg below knee).

c) L5 lesion often due to prolapsed intervertebral disc. Weakness of dorsiflexion *but not eversion* of foot (latter supplied by S1). Ankle jerk is intact, plantar response normal, sensory loss on dorsum of foot often extending to lateral aspect of leg below knee.

Notes

Spastic paraparesis

A common case. You will be asked to examine the legs. You must be able to show the signs with style and polish. Never forget to test for a sensory level and for absence of the abdominal reflexes. Tell the examiners that you would normally ask the patient about bowel and bladder function and test sacral sensation.

If allowed to proceed, you should examine the arms. You may be able to localise the lesion (NB C5/6, absent biceps/supinator jerks, brisk triceps jerk). Ask the examiner's permission to test the neck movements. Again, be ready with your differential diagnosis, which as well as cord compression should include multiple sclerosis, transverse myelitis, subacute combined degeneration of the cord (peripheral neuropathy usually present), anterior spinal artery thrombosis (dorsal columns spared), parasaggital meningioma.

Notes

Wasting of the small muscles of the hand

A popular case ("Examine these hands").

Remember that rheumatoid arthritis and old age are common causes of this. First establish whether the wasting and weakness is *generalised* or whether it is restricted to the muscles supplied by the median or ulnar nerves (test abductor pollucis brevis and interossei). NB combined median and ulnar nerve lesions will of course produce generalised weakness and wasting but this is rare; distal muscular atrophy is another rare peripheral cause.

If the disturbance is generalised the lesion is likely to be *central:* i.e.

* Lesions of the cord affecting T1

  e.g. Motor neurone disease
  Syringomyelia

* Lesions affecting T1 Root

  e.g. Neurofibroma
  Cervical spondylosis (relatively rare at this level)

* Lesions of the brachial plexus affecting T1

  e.g. Klumpke's paralysis
  Cervical ribs
  Pancoast tumour.

You should therefore

* Look for fasciculation in the hand and arm (prominent in motor neurone disease: if you suspect this diagnosis proceed as on p.102) and for wasting and weakness in the rest of the arm.
* Test for loss of reflexes and spinothalamic sensation in the arm (syringomyelia).
* Test sensation over T1 dermatome.
* Palpate for cervical ribs.
* Observe for Horner's syndrome (see p.78).

Notes

Proximal myopathy

The candidate is usually asked to examine the lower limbs neurologically.

Remember the common causes:

* Polymyositis/dermatomyositis (NB tender muscles, rashes, especially on cheeks, eyelids (heliotrope), and over small joints of hands).
* Cushing's syndrome (ask about history of steroid ingestion).
* Thyrotoxicosis (look for goitre, eye signs, rapid pulse, tremor).
* Carcinoma.
* Diabetes (amyotrophy:asymmetrical especially in lower limbs of middle-aged or elderly male non-insulin dependent diabetics).
* Osteomalacia.
* Hereditary muscular dystrophy (see p.106).

Notes

Cerebellar signs

Occasionally you will simply be asked to "Demonstrate some cerebellar signs on this patient". Cerebellar testing may also come up in the context of ataxia or tremor and you must be able to go through a range of tests:

Look for:

1. Intention tremor/past-pointing (dysmetria) in finger-nose test.
2. Oscillation of upper limb in outstretched arm test (*see Bouchier and Morris p. 310*).
3. Dysdiadochokinesia on rapid supination/pronation of wrist and hand-tapping.
4. Lower limb ataxia with heel-shin test.
5. Hypotonia, pendular reflexes.
6. Nystagmus.
7. Scanning dysarthria.
8. Ataxic gait (falls towards affected side) or truncal ataxia.

Revise the causes of cerebellar signs: demyelinating disease is common and should be mentioned early.

Notes

Tremor

You may be asked to look at the hands or to "Examine the arms neurologically". Having found a tremor, you must determine whether it is of resting, postural or intention type. Always test the tone in the arms carefully as this may reveal extrapyramidal rigidity. With postural tremor you should look for signs of thyroid disease and tell the examiner that you would like to know whether there is a family history of tremor and whether the patient is on any medications (e.g. salbutamol, lithium). With an intention tremor, test for other cerebellar signs (see p.93).

Notes

Other dyskinesias

Revise the definitions and causes of chorea, athetosis, dystonia, hemiballismus, myoclonus, tics *(see Medicine International Vol. 1 No 32 PP 1516-1521.).*

Chorea is sometimes shown: remember that drugs (e.g. neuroleptics, L-dopa) are a common cause. 'Senile' chorea is a cause in the elderly. Tell the examiner that you would like to know if there was a family history of the condition (Huntington's chorea or hereditary non-progressive chorea) and that you would like to test the patient's higher cerebral functions (dementia in Huntington's chorea). Ask about previous rheumatic fever and history or oral contraception.

Rare causes worth remembering are polycythaemia rubra vera, thyrotoxicosis and systemic lupus erythematosus.

In younger patients with dyskinesias always check for Kayser-Fleischer rings.

Notes

Dysphasia/Dysarthria

The candidate is asked to "Test this patient's speech", or "Ask this patient a few questions".

Start by asking simple questions, such as "What is your name?", "Where do you live?". You should be able to quickly distinguish between disorders of phonation (dysphonia), articulation (dysarthria, see below) and speech content (dysphasia). The latter is the most common short case.
The essential point is to distinguish between *expressive* and *receptive* dysphasia. In *expressive* (Broca's) aphasia the patient has great difficulty in finding the words with which to reply to your questions. In contrast, if the patient has a sensory aphasia, he will reply fluently to your questions but the speech is often irrelevant or unintelligible with jargon, paraphrasias and neologisms.

Test the patient's ability to name objects (wrist watch, second hand and winder on watch. Difficulity in naming objects is found in both motor and sensory aphasia but is relatively selectively impaired in the rare nominal dysphasia (lesion in angular gyrus).

You must now test for comprehension difficulty (pointing towards sensory aphasia) by asking the patient to perform specific tasks e.g. "Touch your nose", "Pick up the pen".

Ask if you may test for alexia and agraphia (indicating extension of damage to parieto-occipital region. NB May be part of Gerstmann's syndrome, see p.108).

Remember that many patients have features of both sensory and expressive dysphasia.

You may be asked the site of the lesion:

* Broca's area; inferior frontal gyrus of dominant hemisphere.

* Wernicke's area; posterior part of superior temporal gyrus plus adjacent parts of parietal and occipital cortex of dominant hemisphere.

Notes

Dysarthria

Have a selection of tongue-twisters ready to use:

e.g. The Methodist Episcopal Church
Baby hippopotamus
West Register Street

You must be able to recognise the following types of speech:

* Pseudobulbar (monotonous, high-pitched, indistinct 'hot potato' speech). NB. emotional liability and bilateral (though often asymmetrical) pyramidal signs are present in pseudobulbar palsy.

* Bulbar (nasal)

* Cerebellar (scanning or staccato)

* Parkinsonian (slow, slurred, low-pitched, monotonous and quiet)

Remember that poorly-fitting, or absent, dentures are a common cause of dysarthria; it may also occur with seventh nerve palsy (e.g. Bell's palsy).

Notes

Gait

Be able to recognise the gaits listed below and make notes on the signs and causes of each. A popular case is to present the candidate with an ataxic patient: "Watch this patient walk and then examine anything you think relevant". It is important that, as well as testing for cerebellar signs, you remember to perform Romberg's test and to check joint position sense and vibration sense to distinguish sensory from cerebellar ataxia. Parkinsonian gait is not to be confused with the short shuffling steps of 'marche au petit pas' occurring in diffuse cerebrovascular disease.

Fill in the signs and causes *Notes*

Hemiplegic

Paraplegic

Parkinsonism

Sensory ataxia

Cerebellar

Proximal muscle weakness (waddling gait).

Parkinsonism

This may be presented by asking you to observe the face, to watch the patient walking or to examine the arms neurologically.

Mild cog-wheel rigidity may be reinforced by asking the patient to flex and extend one arm while you are testing tone on the other.
Bradykinesia may be elicited by asking the patient to touch his thumb with each of his fingers.

The coarse, pill-rolling tremor (4-6 cps) at rest is characteristic.
Pay careful attention to the patient's gait: note that loss of arm swing is an early feature. Look for flexed posture.

Remember to test for a positive 'glabellar tap'. Look for seborrhoea and excessive sweating and test for dysarthria.

Perform a functional test e.g. ask the patient to undo a button.

If there is time you could add an examination for vertical gaze palsy (Steele-Richardson syndrome) and postural hypotension (marked in Shy-Drager syndrome, but may be iatrogenic e.g. L-dopa treatment).

Notes

Friedreich's ataxia (autosomal recessive)

Pes cavus may again serve as a clue. The patient will have evidence of cerebellar disturbance (see p. 93) often with concurrent evidence of pyramidal weakness in the legs and impairment of dorsal column-mediated sensation. The ankle jerks disappear before the knee jerks: the condition is one of the causes of absent ankle jerks with extensor plantars (see below).

Look for evidence of heart failure (cardiomyopathy) and optic atrophy.

Causes of absent knee jerks with extensor plantars:

- Motor neurone disease
- Diabetes mellitus
- Subacute combined degeneration of the cord
- Neurosyphilis (tabo paresis)
- Friedreich's ataxia
- Conus medullaris lesion.

Remember that a more common cause of mixed cerebellar, pyramidal and dorsal column signs is multiple sclerosis.

Notes

Peroneal muscular atrophy (Charcot-Marie-Tooth disease, autosomal dominant).

Suspect this diagnosis in a patient with pes cavus (also seen in Friedreich's ataxia) and wasting of the peronei, and calf muscles and distal third of the thigh (inverted champagne bottle appearance).

Remember that in contrast to motor neurone disease there is usually evidence of mild sensory loss and absent reflexes and plantar responses in the legs (reflexes in the legs are *usually* brisk in motor neurone disease).

Note that two major forms of the disease are now recognised:

Type I: hypertrophic type, with enlarged peripheral nerves and segmental demyelination;

Type II: neuronal type, no hypertrophic changes; axonal degeneration *(see Medicine International 1983 vol. 1 no. 32 p. 1510 J. E. McLeod.)*

Notes

Motor neurone disease

A very common short case: the candidate is asked to examine either the upper or lower limbs or (occasionally) the cranial nerves/patient's speech.

The importance of *inspection* of limbs is great in this case, fasciculation being missed by candidates moving too hastily to the rest of the examination. It may be brought out by flicking the muscles: do this if you are suspicious of fasciculation. NB *fibrillation* is an *EMG finding* - a common question.

* Remember that there is often a mixture of upper and lower motor neurone signs: commonly the signs in the arms are predominantly of the lower motor neurone type, with mainly upper motor neurone signs in the legs; knee jerks are usually exaggerated.

- * Demonstrate absence of sensory loss, and ask to look at the patient's tongue (for fasciculation).

- * Test the jaw jerk (often exaggerated) and listen to the patient's speech.

- * If allowed to ask questions, ask about difficulty in swallowing.

- * Revise the signs of the three classical forms of presentation (amyotrophic lateral sclerosis, progressive muscular atrophy, progressive bulbar palsy) but remember that these are often present together in the same patient. Note also that progressive bulbar palsy is often combined with upper motor neurone signs (e.g. brisk jaw jerk) and evidence of pseudobulbar palsy *(see Oxford Textbook of Medicine pp. 21-92).*

Syringomyelia

The candidate is often asked to examine the arms. The classical signs will only be brought out if your method of examination is accurate and thorough. The following refers to a classical case.

- * There is a wasting of the upper limbs (including the small hand muscles).

- * Tone is reduced in the upper limb, as is power, especially distally.

- * The reflexes in the arms are reduced or absent.

- * Sensory testing will reveal loss of pain and temperature with preservation of vibration, light touch and joint position sense. These signs are usually asymmetrical (maximal on the same side as the lesion).

Look for evidence of Charcot's joint at the shoulder, which may occur in longstanding cases, and trophic changes in the hands.

Ask the examiner if you may examine the lower limbs (usually pyramidal signs on the side of the lesion). Look for Horner's syndrome and ask whether you may examine the cranial nerves for signs of syringobulbia: loss of pain and temperature sensation on the face (classically progressing forward from behind; sensory loss of the so-called 'onion skin' type); bulbar palsy; nystagmus.

Notes

Tabes dorsalis

Patients with neurosyphilis still appear in the examination. Know the signs of this and of 'general paralysis of the insane' just in case!

Notes

Dystrophia myotonica

A very popular Membership case. The candidate is usually asked to examine the cranial nerves. You must be able to recognise the facial appearance *early (see Parsons, p.190).*

Note:

* Frontal baldness (females may wear a wig.)
* Expressionless face and smooth forehead despite ptosis. NB in tabes dorsalis there is a bilateral ptosis with *overactive* frontalis muscle.
* Wasting of temporalis and masseters (producing 'hatchet' face) and sternomastoids.
* Bilateral ptosis and facial muscle weakness.
* Cataracts.

Test for the myotonic hand shake. Ask if you may:

a) test limb muscles for weakness and wasting (especially distally)

b) observe for gynaecomastia and testicular atrophy

c) test higher intellectual function (IQ often low and dementia may occur).

Other abnormalities which may occur are diabetes mellitus, cardiomyopathy, respiratory infections (muscular difficulties + IgG deficiency) and disordered oesophageal and bowel motility.

Notes

Muscular dystrophy

Revise the appearance, inheritance and prognosis of the following types *(see Patten pp.184-186)* and expand the following chart:

TYPE	FEATURES	IQ	PROGNOSIS
SEVERE X-LINKED DUCHENNE (uncommon as a short case)	Presents 3rd year of life severe proximal weakness of lower limbs Calf hypertrophy Ankle jerks preserved Cardiac muscle affected Onset 5th-25th year	May be low	Death towards end of second decade
BENIGN X-LINKED BECKER TYPE MUSCULAR DYSTROPHY	Weakness and wasting of pelvic and shoulder-girdle muscles	Normal	Many survive to normal age
FACIO SCAPULO-HUMERAL DYSTROPHY (Autosomal Dominant)	Onset often in adolescence Facial weakness: ptosis Difficulty in closing eyes Wasting of sternomastoids spinati pectorals triceps biceps Marked scapular winging Occasionally deltoids hypertrophy	Normal	Normal life span
LIMB GIRDLE MUSCULAR DYSTROPHY (Autosomal recessive)	Onset usually in second or third decade. Weakness and wasting may begin in either shoulder or pelvic girdle muscles. Hypertrophy of calves and/or deltoids may occur. Ankle jerks preserved	Normal	Often severely disabled by middle life with death before normal age

Note: a scapuloperoneal muscular dystrophy may occur, which may be a myopathy, a neuropathy, a form of spinal atrophy or a combination of these. *(see Parsons p.170.).*

Stroke

Patients with straightforward strokes are sometimes shown as short cases. The candidate may be asked to "Assess this patient who has had a stroke", or to "Examine the limbs". You should be able to demonstrate the signs quickly and efficiently.

Hemiplegia

Having elicited the signs in the limbs, test for sensory inattention, visual inattention and hemianopia, and ask if you may test the patient's speech. Show that you are considering the aetiology by feeling the patient's pulse (? atrial fibrillation), auscultating for valve lesions and carotid bruits and taking the patient's blood pressure.

Revise the signs of parietal lobe dysfunction as these are occasionally asked (see table).

Pariental lobe signs

1. **Either hemisphere**

   * Loss of accurate localisation of touch, joint position sense and temperature appreciation (*see Patten p. 73*). N.B. parietal drift in outstretched arm test.
   * Loss of two-point discrimination
   * Astereognosis
   * Dysgraphaesthesia
   * Sensory inattention
   * Sometimes: attention hemianopia, homonymous hemianopia or lower quadrantic hemianopia.

2. **Dominant parietal lobe**

   Additional features:

   * Receptive dysphasia
   * Gerstmann's syndrome (if lesion in angular gyrus):

     dysgraphia + dyslexia
     dyscalculia
     left-right disorientation
     finger agnosia
     ideomotor apraxia may be associated.

   * Bilateral ideomotor apraxia (unable to imitate gestures)
   * Bilateral ideational apraxia (failure to execute composite actions: e.g. lighting a match when given closed box).

3. **Non-dominant parietal lobe**

   * Dressing apraxia
   * Constructional apraxia
   * Hemiasomatognosia (loss of appreciation of opposite side of body) or neglect of opposite side.

Notes

Lateral medullary syndrome

Revise the signs of this syndrome (due to posterior inferior cerebellar artery thrombosis) which occasionally appears in the examination *(see Burton p. 113)*.

Notes

DERMATOLOGICAL SHORT CASES

Dermatological short cases

It is common to be shown skin lesions in the Membership examination.

Many are 'spot' diagnoses but others may be more difficult and if unsure you should give a differential diagnosis. In all cases you must give a clear, accurate description of the lesion using recognised dermatological terms, the meaning of which you must understand.

Few candidates will have worked in this specialty so it is wise to arrange to sit in on some dermatology clinics before the clinical. If possible, on these occasions, practise describing each patient's lesions to the consultant and making your own diagnosis before he tells you what it is. You will rapidly become familiar with the terminology and the appearance of the common lesions.

The following is a list of terms which you should be able to use accurately.

Dermatological terms

Erythema	:	Redness due to increased skin perfusion.
Macule	:	A flat, circumscribed area of discoloration.
Papule	:	A circumscribed elevation of the skin less than 1 cm in diameter.
Nodule	:	A palpable mass larger than 1 cm in diameter.
Plaque	:	A flat topped palpable disc shaped lesion.
Vesicle	:	A circumscribed fluid containing elevation less than 5 mm in diameter.
Bulla	:	A blister more than 5 mm in diameter.
Pustule	:	A visible accumulation of free pus.
Weal	:	An area of dermal oedema; usually transient, raised, white, compressible, with a pink margin.
Scale	:	A flake of easily-detached keratin.
Crust	:	An accumulation of dried exudate.
Excoriation	:	A shallow abrasion due to scratching.
Lichenification	:	Areas of increased epidermal thickness and accentuated skin markings secondary to chronic rubbing.
Sclerosis	:	Induration of the dermis or subcutaneous tissues.
Purpura	:	Discoloration of the skin or mucosa due to extravasation of red cells. NB Does not blanch on pressure.

Petechiae	:	Small purpuric lesions (less than 2 mm in diameter).
Ecchymosis	:	A large extravasation of blood.
Telangiectasia	:	Permanently dilated, visible small vessels.
Ulcer	:	An excavation due to loss of tissue, including the epidermal surface.

Notes

Eczema

Remember the cardinal signs: erythema, papules, vesicles, hyperkeratosis with scaling, exudation of serum (weeping) and crusting. Excoriations and lichenification may be present.

Revise and make notes on the different types of eczema listed below:

Exogenous	:	Primary irritant Allergic
Endogenous	:	Atopic Seborrhoeic Gravitational (varicose) Asteatotic Discoid (nummular) Pompholyx on hand and foot

Be ready to discuss the treatment of eczema in both the acute and chronic forms.

Notes

Psoriasis

This is a common short case. Remember the classical description: raised, red, circular or oval plaques with sharply marginated edges and a scaly surface.

Look for involvement in the commonest sites first, to show that you are familiar with these:

* extensor aspect of knees and elbows
* sacral area
* scalp (especially behind the ears)

Proceed to look for nail changes:

* thimble-pitting

* onycholysis (occasionally with green discoloration due to chromogenic bacteria). Other causes include trauma, fungal infection and thyrotoxicosis.

* thickening and ridging of the nail-plate.

Look for evidence of arthropathy in both the small (especially distal interphalangeal) and large joints (see psoriatic arthropathy p.130).

Remember the variants which may occur:

guttate
pustular
flexural
erythrodermic.

As with eczema it is not uncommon to be asked to give a brief account of the treatment of psoriasis and you should revise this carefully.
(see Burton pp.15-17).

Notes

Lichen planus

This is occasionally used as a *spot diagnosis* case. You must be able to recognise the classical purplish, flat-topped, shiny, polygonal papules.

* Look for Wickham's striae over the lesions.

* Show that you are aware of the common distribution by looking especially at the flexor aspects of the wrists, trunk and lower limbs.

* Look for lesions in the mouth (found in 25% of cases).

* Look for nail changes: pits, ridges, splits or even complete nail loss.

* Ask if you may take a drug history (e.g. chloroquine and gold may cause a lichen planus-like reaction).

Remember that, like psoriasis and warts, lichen planus exhibits Koebner's phenomenon (occurring in sites of scratching or other injury).

Notes

Rosacea

You will be asked to "Look at the patient's face". You must be able to recognise the characteristic lesions: papules, pustules, erythema and telangiectasia over the cheeks, nose, forehead and chin.

You must look carefully for eye complications: usually keratitis but occasionally blepharitis, conjunctivitis, iritis and even episcleritis.

Revise the treatment of the condition *(see Fry).*

Some candidates confuse this with the butterfly rash of SLE. Remember that in the latter condition there are no papules or pustules, but unlike rosacea, there may be scaling and follicular plugging.

Notes

Pityriasis rosea

Remember that the lesions are usually *oval* and occur on the trunk, macules tending to be aligned along the skin creases. Look for a 'herald patch' on the trunk and check lesions for centripetal scaling.

Notes

Lupus erythematosus

A. Systemic

Butterfly rash is a common spot diagnosis ("Look at the face").

* Look for a symmetrical rash with erythema, scaling, telangiectasia and follicular plugging. Chronic lesions may show hyperpigmentation and atrophy.

* Inspect other areas exposed to sunlight, especially arms, for rash.

* Look for evidence of oral ulceration (present in 30% of cases).

Before proceeding further, it may be as well to state the diagnosis and the signs. You should then ask the examiner if you may examine:

a) the scalp for alopecia
b) the hands for: erythema of thenar or hypothenar areas
dilated nail-fold capillaries, periungual
infarcts and splinter haemorrhages

c) The elbows and knees for erythema, telangiectasia and scaling.

You may ask if you may take a drug history *(e.g. hydrallazine: see BMJ 289, 410, 1984).*

Remember that other rashes may occur in SLE, e.g. livedo reticularis, urticaria, purpura due to thrombocytopenia, vasculitic rashes, pyoderma gangrenosum.

You are unlikely to be asked to proceed to general examination in the short cases but you should have a scheme for doing so just in case.

Notes

B. **Discoid**

The scaly red plaques with follicular plugging may be shown as a short case. As well as on the face (the most common site) look for lesions on the scalp (there may be scarring alopecia), ears, neck and hands.
Look for crusting and erosions of the lips.

Remember that scarring is more a feature of discoid than of systemic lupus and you should comment on this if it is present.

You may be asked about the relationship of discoid LE to the systemic form: remember that only 5% of cases of discoid LE convert to the systemic form, whereas up to 33% of cases of SLE have discoid-type lesions at some time during the course of the disease *(see Rook, Wilkinson, Ebling, p19).*

Notes

Xanthomata

These are commonly shown as a spot diagnosis case, which you should recognise immediately and go on to look for associations. The following is a simplified guide. You must be fully conversant with the classification, investigation and treatment of hyperlipidaemia *(see, for example, Medicine International 14, pp.580-589, 1985 J., Mann, M. Ball.)*

A. **Tendon xanthomata**

The candidate may be asked to "Look at these hands." Tendon xanthomata classically occur in the extensor tendons and may become more obvious when the patient clenches his fist.

Look also for xanthomata in the Achilles tendons and patellar tendons.

Look for xanthelasmata and corneal arcus.

Remember that tendon xanthomata are classically found in Type IIA lipoproteinaemia: this may be *primary* (familial hypercholesterolaemia), or *secondary* (seen in jaundice).

B. **Xanthelasmata**

This time the candidate may be invited to "Examine the eyes". Never forget the importance of inspection. Look for corneal arcus, which often coexists with xanthelasmata and is typically most pronounced at the 12 and 6 o'clock positions (in contrast to corneal calcification which tends to be maximal at the 3 and 9 o'clock positions).

Look for tendon xanthomas in the hands and Achilles tendons (see above). Check the palms for xanthomata (see D below) and tell the examiners that you would like to take the patient's blood pressure and test the urine for glucose (hypertension and diabetes mellitus being associated with Type IIB lipoproteinaemia).

Remember that xanthelasmata and corneal arcus may occur in:

a) normal people
b) Type IIA lipoproteinaemia (see A above)
c) Type IIB lipoproteinaemia (mixed hyperlipidaemia)
d) Type III lipoproteinaemia.

C. **Eruptive xanthomata**

You should be able to recognise the multiple red or yellow vesicles which are found on extensor surfaces: back, buttocks, elbows, knees. These are not usually associated with tendon xanthomata or xanthelasmata.

Ask if you may inspect the fundi for lipaemia retinalis (found in severe hyperlipidaemia) and test the urine for glucose.

Eruptive xanthomata classically occur in lipoproteinaemia Type IV (familial hypertriglyceridaemia), which may be associated with diabetes mellitus and obesity. It also occurs in Types I and V lipoproteinaemia.

D. **Palmar xanthomata**

These rare xanthomata could also be shown as a spot diagnosis case, the orange or yellow discolourations of the palmar and digital creases being most distinctive. Look also for 'tubo-eruptive xanthomata' characteristically found over the knees and elbows.

Check the eyelids for xanthelasmata, which are also associated.

Palmar and tubo-eruptive xanthomata strongly suggest the presence of remnant hyperlipoproteinaemia (Type III).

Notes

Bullous disorders

Revise the features and associations of the following rashes which occasionally occur as short cases:

Dermatitis herpetiformis: look for characteristic distribution on extensor surface of elbows, knees and on occiput, interscapular and gluteal regions.

Pemphigus: lesions in mouth common. Bullae tend to break easily. Widespread crusting and erosions.

Phemphigoid: mucosal ulceration rare. Tense bullae present with erythematous plaques.

Erythema multiforme: pleomorphic eruption (macules, papules, bullae). Look for target lesions and for lesions in the mouth. NB Stevens-Johnson syndrome, a severe form with fever, arthralgia, orogenital and conjunctival involvement.
(see Fry)

Notes

Neurofibromatosis

Be able to demonstrate the various skin lesions (fibromata, plexiform neurofibromata, cafe-au-lait spots, axillary freckles) and have a scheme for general examination, e.g. check hearing (acoustic neuroma), visual acuity and fundi (optic glioma), look for kyphoscoliosis, ask to check blood pressure (phaeochromocytoma).

Revise the other complications.

Notes

Adenoma sebaceum

Know the other skin manifestations of tuberose sclerosis: 'ash leaf' depigmented macules on trunk; 'shagreen patch' on lower trunk; periungual fibromata. Ask if you may inspect fundi for phakomata.

Other associations: lung and kidney hamartomas, cardiac rhabdomyoma, polycystic kidneys, cerebral glioma (patient may have craniotomy scar). Epilepsy and mental retardation are other features.

Notes

Lupus pernio

A rare short case. Other skin manifestations of sarcoidosis: erythema nodosum (in acute form of disease), scar infiltration, granuloma of nose, brownish nodules (micropapular sarcoid), sarcoid plaques of limbs, shoulders, buttocks, thighs *(see Oxford Textbook of Medicine p.20-90).*

Notes

Lesions on the legs

Necrobiosis lipoidica diabeticorum

A common 'spot' case. Associated with diabetes in about 75% of cases; the related granuloma annulare *(Oxford Textbook of Medicine p.20-91)* is much less predictably associated. Revise the histology of these lesions (occasionally asked): collagen degeneration with surrounding epithelioid and giant cells.

Pretibial myxoedema

Remember to check for thyroid acropachy, exophthalmos/ocular palsies, goitre/thyroidectomy scar.

Erythema nodosum

Revise the causes: streptococcal sore throat, sarcoidosis, drugs, viral and chlamydial infection and tuberculosis are the commonest causes in Britain today but remember that Crohn's disease and ulcerative colitis are common associations in teaching hospital practice. You are likely to be asked how you would investigate the case.

Notes

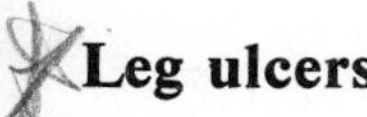

Leg ulcers

The three common forms are:

1. Venous ulceration: usually over medial malleolus; gently sloping edge; may be eczema surrounding the area with pigmentation, sclerosis (atrophie blanche).
2. Ischaemic: *painful* punched out ulcer: commonly on toes dorsum of feet, shins and around malleoli.
3. Neuropathic: *painless* punched out ulcer often on soles of feet or heels. (e.g. diabetes, spina bifida). Charcot's arthropathy may be present. NB In diabetes, ischaemia and neuropathy often both contribute to ulceration often with superadded infection.

Examination:

After describing the ulcer, look for signs of poor peripheral perfusion and test the peripheral pulses. If you suspect neuropathic ulcer (commonly shown) test for sensory neuropathy and say that you would like to test the patient's urine for sugar.

Remember that an everted edge occurs in squamous cell carcinoma e.g. Marjolin's ulcer.

In a negroid patient do not forget the possibility of sickle cell anaemia. Ulcers also occur with hereditary spherocytosis.

Other rarer causes to bear in mind include vasculitis in systemic lupus erythematosus (look for butterfly rash) and rheumatoid arthritis (especially with Felty's syndrome).

A special case, also occurring on the trunk, buttocks, upper limbs and face, is pyoderma gangrenosum, an irregular ulcer with an overhanging purple edge and necrotic base.

Causes of pyoderma gangrenosum:

* Inflammatory bowel disease (especially ulcerative colitis).
* Benign monoclonal gammopathy.
* Rheumatoid arthritis.
* Leukaemia.

Rare causes of ulcers include gumma, tuberculosis, hypertension (Marterell's ulcer).

Notes

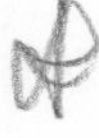

Leg oedema

A common case. Look to see whether the oedema is unilateral or bilateral. Test for pitting. Look for sacral oedema. *Non-pitting oedema* may occur with 'lipoedema' due to long-standing oedema of any cause, but remember Milroy's disease (primary lymphoedema), which is often asymmetrical. (Filariasis may cause a similar picture).

In **bilateral oedema** look for:

* Signs of right heart failure, especially raised jugular venous pressure.

* Involvement of the face/periorbital tissues suggests nephrotic syndrome (ask to test patient's urine for protein).

* Signs of chronic liver disease (hypoalbuminaemia may occur, look especially for leuconychia).

* Palpate inguinal nodes for enlargement; malignant infiltration may cause secondary lymphoedema.

* Comment on the desirability of abdominal, rectal and vaginal examination to exclude malignancy. Remember that bilateral iliac vein thrombosis may cause bilateral oedema, as may pregnancy.

In **unilateral oedema** look for

* Other signs of deep venous thrombosis.
* Measure the calf with a tape-measure.
* Look for varicose veins, venous eczema and ulceration.

An important differential diagnosis of calf swelling is a ruptured Baker's cyst; consider this especially in a patient with osteoarthritis or rheumatoid arthritis (a common discussion point). Ultrasound, arthrography and/or venography may be required to distinguish between the two conditions, which may even coexist. Milroy's disease must again be considered in the differential.

Finally note that cellulitis may produce inflammatory oedema as well as lymphatic oedema due to lymphangitis; look for the latter as well as lymphadenopathy in the inguinal region.

Notes

Hereditary haemorrhagic telangiectasia

More often shown as a slide in the written section but occasionally used as a short case. "Look at this patient's face." Look for telangiectases not only on the face and lips but also on the conjunctivae and in the mouth. Look also for involvement of the fingers. You may be allowed to ask questions (family history, GI bleeding, etc.). Revise the complications.

Notes

Purpura

Occasionally shown as a short case: revise the causes; remember that these fall largely into 2 groups:

1) Vessel disorders 2) Platelet disorders

See Thompson, chapter 24. Note that congulation disorders tend to produce large ecchymoses rather than purpura.

You should:

a) Observe the distribution of the lesions, e.g.

 * Senile purpura/steroids often affect backs of hands and forearms.

 * Henoch Schonlein purpura classically appears over lower limbs and buttocks.

 * Scurvy over lower limbs/backs of thighs with perifollicular haemorrhages plus corkscrew hairs; look for swollen gums (other causes of gum hypertrophy: phenytoin, monocytic leukaemia).

b) Inspect: *palate* for petechial haemorrhages
 gums for ulceration and haemorrhage (suggests neutropenia and thrombocytopenia of e.g. leukaemia).

c) Inspect conjunctivae and fundi for haemorrhages (fundal haemorrhages only in *severe* thrombocytopenia).

d) Look for evidence of cause:

 * ? cushingoid (ask for history of steroid ingestion).
 * ? rheumatoid arthritis, systemic lupus erythematosus, infective endocarditis. Note that vasculitic lesions tend to be discrete, raised and polychromatic
 * ? chronic liver disease (thrombocytopenia may occur though coagulopathy due to hypoprothrombinaemia is more common).
 * ? elastic skin/hyperextensible joints (Ehlers-Danlos syndrome).

Ask if you may examine for enlargement of liver, spleen or nodes. (NB spleen is often impalpable or only just palpable in idiopathic thrombocytopenic purpura, a common cause).

Remember to include disseminated intravascular coagulation (e.g. due to meningococcal septicaemia) in your differential diagnosis.

Revise the signs of Moschowitz's syndrome, a popular examination question.

Notes

Vitiligo

Occasionally shown as a discussion case: revise the associations and modes of treatment.

Acanthosis nigricans

Another spot diagnosis: look for characteristic distribution: axillae, groins, umbilicus, nipples. You will be asked the associations:

- Obesity
- Internal malignancy (usually adenocarcinoma)
- Endocrine causes:
  - diabetes mellitus
  - Cushing's syndrome
  - acromegaly
  - polycystic ovary syndrome
  - congenital partial lipodystrophy (see p.141)

Notes

RHEUMATOLOGICAL SHORT CASES

Revise your method of examining large joints, especially the hip, knee and ankle joints, as you will occasionally be asked to do this in the clinical. Be sure that you can examine the spine and sacroiliac joints proficiently.

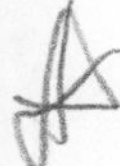

Rheumatoid arthritis

Usually you will be asked to "Examine these hands" (see p.28).

Although this is unlikely as a short case be prepared to look for evidence of systemic complications (especially ocular, cardiac, pulmonary and neurological) and devise a scheme for doing this rapidly.

Felty's syndrome occasionally occurs as a short case, the candidate being asked to palpate the abdomen (where he should find splenomegaly).

Notes

Ankylosing spondylitis

Be sure to revise your methods of examining the spine and sacroiliac joints during your preparation for the clinical.

Advanced cases may have the classic 'question mark' spine, with thoracic kyphosis, hyperextension of the neck and loss of lumbar lordosis. Chest expansion may be limited due to fusion of the costovertebral joints.

Examine the spine: in early cases (patient is typically a young m[illegible] restriction of movement in the lumbar spine especially lateral flexion but also forward flexion. This may be gauged by measuring the increase in distance between two fingers placed on the top and bottom of the lumbar spine while holding a tape measure: the distance should 'expand' by over 5 cm on forward flexion. There may also be diminution of rotation (thoracic spine involvement) and flattening of the lumbar lordosis.

Test for sacroiliac pain: use several methods but always include 'springing the pelvis' and pushing the flexed knee towards the opposite shoulder (watch the patient's face and be careful not to cause excessive pain while doing this).

Measure chest expansion: less than 2cm is pathological.

Look for:

a) peripheral arthropathy, especially large joints e.g. Knees, ankles (10%)
b) tenderness over Achilles tendons (tendonitis)
c) iritis (20%)

Ask the examiner if you may:

1) Examine heart for aortic regurgitation (1%)
2) Examine lungs for apical fibrosis (1%)

Notes

Reiter's disease:

The patient is usually a young male. Remember that although the arthritis is usually polyarticular the diagnosis must be considered when a patient presents just with a large swollen knee joint (see p.133).

After examining affected joints, test for sacroiliac tenderness, (sacroiliitis in 20% of cases) and for tenderness over the Achilles tendons and plantar fascia. Look for keratoderma blennorhagica on the soles and palms and for evidence of conjunctivitis or iritis (the latter occurs with repeated attacks).

Look in the mouth for ulcers and tell the examiner that you would like to inspect the genitalia for circinate balanitis.

Tell the examiner that you would like to know whether the patient has any history of urethral discharge (chlamydial infection) or diarrhoea (Salmonella, Shigella, Yersinia, Campylobacter).

Notes

Psoriatic arthropathy

A popular case. The distal arthropathy of the hands is often presented. Thimble-pitting of the nails and plaques of psoriasis at the elbow or elsewhere should not escape your attention.

Remember the 5 different forms of psoriatic arthropathy:

1. Asymmetrical distal interphalangeal joint involvement (usually with nail changes).
2. Seronegative rheumatoid-like pattern.
3. Oligoarthritis.
4. Arthritis mutilans.
5. Ankylosing spondylitis-like pattern.

Notes

Scleroderma

A common short case ("Look at these hands"). Look for the characteristic skin features in the hands:

* Thickening and tightening of the skin which may appear shiny (dermal atrophy). Early cases show only oedema.

* Subcutaneous calcification (usually localised to finger tips but may involve extensor aspects of forearms or elbows). Occasionally widespread, Thibierge-Weissenbach syndrome.

* Ulceration over bony eminences and calcific deposits (look especially at finger-tips).

* There may be areas of increased pigmentation and/or vitiligo.

* Look for polyarthropathy (25%, though arthralgia is much more common) in small joints which may mimic rheumatoid arthritis.

* Look at the face for microstomia with radiating fissures and telangiectases on cheeks and lip margins.
* Look for alopecia which may occur. If allowed to ask questions enquire about Raynaud's phenomenon and dysphagia. Revise the systemic complications.

Occasionally *morphoea* may be shown; revise the appearance.

Notes

Gout

Acute gout is unlikely to be shown unless there is a classical case on the ward. Chronic tophaceous gout may appear, however, the usual case being the asymmetrical arthropathy of the hands.

Remember to look for tophi in the periarticular tissues, bursae (especially olecranon bursa), tendon sheaths, and helices of the ears.

Notes

Painful swollen knee joint

Practise your methods of demonstrating fluid within the joint. Watch the patient while doing this and be careful not to hurt him/her.

Be ready with a list of causes. You may find it useful to expand the following list:

Trauma	
Infections:	septic arthritis gonococcal or meningococcal infection rheumatic fever viral infections
Seronegative arthropathies:	Reiter's disease reactive arthropathy ankylosing spondylitis psoriatic arthropathy enteropathic arthropathy
Metabolic:	gout pseudogout (associated with hyperparathyroidism, hyperuricaemia and gout, haemochromatosis, acromegaly, diabetes mellitus, renal failure, Wilson's disease, ochronosis.)
Haematological:	haemophilia sickle cell anaemia
Osteoarthritis	
Rheumatoid disease	

When discussing your management always mention the importance of aspiration of the joint and culture of the fluid for bacterial infection/ microscopy for crystals.

Notes

ENDOCRINE/METABOLIC CASES

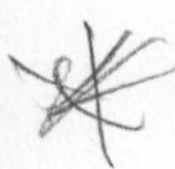

Cushing's syndrome

The candidate is usually asked to "Look at the patient's face". The typical moon-face is usually striking. There may be plethora (polycythaemia), hirsutism and acne.

Look for

* Truncal obesity, interscapular fat accumulation (buffalo hump) and thin legs.
* Purple striae on the abdomen, around the shoulders and breasts and on the thighs. (Striae gravidarum are typically silvery.)
* Evidence of easy bruising, and kyphosis (collapse of osteoporotic vertebrae).

Test muscle power at shoulders and hips for evidence of proximal myopathy. Tell the examiners that you would like to measure the patient's blood pressure and test the urine for sugar, and that you would like to know whether he (or she) is taking steroids.

Notes

Thyroid disease

See the suggested scheme for examination of the thyroid (p. 32). Modify this to suit your own taste and practise it until you can perform it smoothly and rapidly.

Practise palpating different goitres. The firm, rubbery goitre of Hashimoto's thyroiditis is a common case. Occasionally 'classical' patients with the triad of thyroid acropachy, pretibial myxoedema and thyroid eye disease appear in the examination. Always look for these.

Patients with solitary nodules may also appear. You may be asked how you would investigate any of these cases.

Notes

Addidson's disease

The candidate is asked to look at a patient with generalised hyperpigmentation.

Look quickly for classical predominance of hyperpigmentation in:

a) Exposed areas.
b) Friction areas (under straps or rings).
c) Hand creases.

Now inspect the lips, gums and buccal mucosa for pigmented areas.

If the patient is undressed look for adrenalectomy scar (Nelson's syndrome).

Remember that vitiligo may occur in association with Addison's disease, producing a very characteristic picture of areas of both increased and decreased pigmentation.

You may be invited to ask the patient some questions: ask about any history of fatigue, anorexia, weight loss, nausea, abdominal pain or diarrhoea.

Revise the list of causes of diffuse hyperpigmentation *(see Burton p.192).* Remember other causes of raised ACTH (Nelson's syndrome, ectopic ACTH). Popular examination causes included uraemia (clues are anaemia + brown line on nails +/– presence of AV fistula on arms), haemochromatosis (see p. 72), primary biliary cirrhosis (typically middle-aged lady with prominent scratch marks + xanthelasmata) and *porphyria cutanea tarda*. Clues in the latter are scarring on face, neck, forearms, hands, +/- increased skin fragility, erythema, vesicles, bullae, hirsutism. Alcohol related liver disease commonly associated; urinary uroporphyrins raised, especially in attacks; similar skin changes may occur in variegate porphyria.

Notes

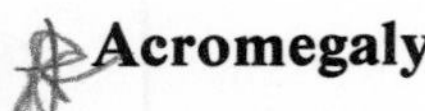

Acromegaly

The candidate is usually asked to look at either the hands or face.

Look for and be ready to comment on the typical features: large hands with broad, spatulate fingers, large lips and nose, prominent supraorbital ridges, protrusion of the lower jaw (prognathism). Look at the skin for evidence of seborrhoea, excessive sweating, acne or hirsuties.

Ask to see the patient's tongue (it may be enlarged, with impressions formed by teeth on the edges), and ask him to clench his teeth; look for dental malocclusion. Note: other causes of large tongue are amyloidosis (primary), cretinism, mongolism.

Now proceed (with examiner's permission) to test for bitemporal hemianopia and optic atrophy. Look for kyphosis (vertebral enlargement occurs) and test for carpal tunnel syndrome.

Tell the examiner that you would like to measure the patient's blood pressure (elevated in 15%) and test the urine for glucose (diabetes mellitus in 10%, impaired glucose tolerance in 20%).

Other signs which could be looked for include enlargement of the thyroid, heart, liver and spleen, and presence of arthropathy of large joints (due to degenerative arthropathy and/or chondrocalanosis).
Gynaecomastia and/or galactorrhoea may also occur.

Always say that you would like to see old photographs of the patient (these are often brought along specially).

Notes

Paget's disease

You will usually be presented with a 'bowed tibia'. Bowing may be anterior and laterally (NB Lateral bowing occurs in rickets, forward bowing (sabre tibia) in syphilis.) Palpate the bone for increased temperature.

Look at the patient's head for the typical skull appearance. After checking for skeletal changes elsewhere, you may ask if you may look for complications such as deafness, optic atrophy or angioid streaks, cardiac failure (high output), cord compression (due to basilar invagination), root lesions due to vertebral damage. Other complications include fractures, immobilisation hypercalcaemia, sarcomatous changes (1-2%), osteoarthritis of related joints.

Notes

Marfan's syndrome (autosomal dominant)

You will usually be asked to look at the patient's hands. Once you have made a diagnosis, be ready to continue with a prepared scheme of examination: check for a high arched palate, lens dislocation (upwards) aortic regurgitation and mitral valve prolapse. (Remember dissecting aneurysm is also associated.) Look for scoliosis.

Note that in homocystinuria (which also causes arachnodactyly) there is mental retardation, *downward* lens dislocation, vascular thromboses, osteoporosis and homocystine in the urine *(see Oxford Textbook of Medicine 1983 p.17.27).*

Notes

Klinefelter's syndrome

Revise the features of this condition. Remember that the patient with the classical form will have eunuchoidal proportions (span more than 5 cm greater than height; sole to symphysis pubis greater than symphysis pubis to crown); patients are generally tall. *(see Hall, Evered and Greene p.104)*

The testes are small and firm (ask permission from both patient and examiners before examining these) and there is a varying degree of hypogonadism; look for poor muscular development and diminished facial, axillary and pubic hair growth.

Gynaecomastia is usually present (you should check that true gynaecomastia is present and not just fat deposition). Revise the other causes of gynaecomastia; commoner causes include:

Drugs (e.g. spironolactone, oestrogens, digitalis, cimetidine)
Hepatic cirrhosis (especially alcoholic)
Bronchial carcinoma
Testicular teratoma
Paraplegia

Revise the rarer causes and have a scheme for investigation of gynaecomastia *(see Prout and Cooper, Chapter 27)*.

Notes

Pseudohypoparathyroidism

On rare occasions this may be shown as a short case. You may be asked to look at the hands (short or absent fourth metacarpal). Learn the features just in case.

Notes

Partial lipodystrophy

A rare short case. There is loss of subcutaneous fat from the face and arms.

The condition is associated with mesangiocapillary glomerulonephritis.

Notes

GENERAL APPROACH QUESTIONS

Occasionally you may be told that a patient has a particular condition (e.g. hypertension) and invited to ask the patient some questions and examine anything which you think is relevant. Although these are unusual short cases, it is worth being prepared for them, this being good general revision.

Examples: This patient has:

a) Hypertension

b) Diabetes mellitus — "Would you ask him some questions/ examine him".

c) Jaundice

d) Renal failure

Make notes on your approach below.

a) Hypertension (a young patient may be shown).

b) Diabetes mellitus

c) Jaundice

d) Renal failure

e) Young stroke

7 : THE EXAMINATION DAY

The clinical part of the Membership examination is held in a variety of centres and it is worth spending some time planning how you will get to your particular hospital. Amazingly, there are always candidates who arrive late, sweating profusely and gasping for breath after running up several flights of stairs. It is impossible to appear suitably composed when in this state. Your body may be ready for fight or flight but neither of these is suitable behaviour in the Membership!

Arrive, therefore, in plenty of time: *at least* half an hour before the starting time. You will be given some forms to fill in and can also use the extra time to smarten yourself up and to check that your instruments are arranged in your pockets so that you can find them without fumbling.

You must pay careful attention to your appearance in the examination.

It is advisable to dress conservatively. For men a dark suit and white shirt, a plain (not club) tie and dark shoes are appropriate; hair should be short. Women should also opt for sober and sensible clothes.

Smell should be neutral: spicey food and alcohol should be avoided for at least a day before the examination.

You will meet three pairs of examiners. Each pair sometimes includes both a more aggressive and a more benign examiner. In any case each examiner will spend an equal proportion of the allotted time with you.

The golden rule is to be polite and courteous at all times. Even if you feel that you are being harassed you must not appear upset or argue: you will achieve nothing by doing this. If one examiner seems to be adopting a rather aggressive approach the other may be sympathetic towards you and it is well known for candidates to pass even after a difficult time. In fact you will often receive little or no feed-back on whether what you are saying is right or wrong, but you must not let this put you off.

Another trap to avoid is that of being pushed into changing your mind over a diagnosis or fact about which you are reasonably certain.
Examiners who ask "Are you sure?" are by no means always implying that you are wrong.

This is completely different from the situation in which an examiner tells you that something you have said is wrong. Never argue in this situation, even if you think you are right.

It is easy to give stupid answers when under pressure. If you do this and realise it then be sure to retract the statement at once and say that you know that it was wrong. This is much better than letting the examiners think that you are totally incompetent.

As mentioned in chapter 2, if you know nothing about a topic about which you are being asked you should admit this at once to avoid wasting time or giving an answer which is false or dangerous.

Try to think positively at all stages of the examination. It is your show and every minute must be spent in trying to convince the examiners that you will be a worthy member of their College. There is very little time in which to do this and you must give maximum concentration to the task for the whole period of the examination. The candidate who appears fully alert is more likely to capture the examiners' attention.
They will know more than you about their own subject and you may well learn something during the examination. You are not expected to be a specialist yet.

Finally, it is sometimes claimed that there is a large element of luck in how you get on in the clinical. This tends to be exaggerated, particularly by those who fail. If you have prepared carefully and thoroughly, the dice will be loaded heavily in your favour.

BIBLIOGRAPHY

The following books are referred to in the text by the name of the author(s):

Burton, J. L. **Aids to Postgraduate Medicine.** 5th edition 1988. Churchill Livingstone.

Burton, J. L. **Essentials of Dermatology.** 3rd edition 1990. Churchill Livingstone.

Chester, E. **Schrires Clinical Cardiology.** 4th edition 1981. John Wright.

Flenley, D. C. **Respiratory Medicine.** 2nd edition 1990. Bailliere Tindall.

Fry, L. **Dermatology: an illustrated guide.** 3rd edition 1983. Update Books.

Gabriel, R. **Postgraduate Nephrology.** 3rd edition 1986. Butterworths.

Hall, R. Evered, D. **A Colour Atlas of Endocrinology.** 2nd edition 1989. Wolfe Medical Publications Ltd.

Kritzinger, E. E. Wright, B. E. **A Colour Atlas of the Eye and Systemic Disease.** 1984. Wolfe Medical Publications Ltd.

Parsons, M. **A Colour Atlas of Clinical Neurology.** 1983. Wolfe Medical Publications Ltd.

Patten, J. **Neurological Differential Diagnosis.** 1977. Harold Starke Ltd.

Prout, B. Cooper, J. **An Outline of Clinical Diagnosis.** 2nd edition 1987. John Wright.

Rook, A. Wilkinson, D. S. Ebling, F. J. G. **Textbook of Dermatology.** 3rd edition 1986. Blackwell Scientific Publications.

Sherlock, S. **Disease of the Liver and Biliary System.** 8th edition 1989. Blackwell Scientific Publications.

Thompson, R. B. **A Short Textbook of Haematology.** 6th edition 1984. Pitman Medical.

Weatherall, D. J. Ledingham, J. C. G. Warrell, D. A. **Oxford Textbook of Medicine.** 2nd edition 1987. Oxford University Press.

INDEX

MRCP PART 2 PREPARATION FOR THE CLINICAL EXAMINATION